Fat Loss Stability

How the Body Regulates Stored Energy, Adaptation, and Long-Term Change

Nathan Reed

PERENNIAL PUBLISHING

Published by Perennial Publishing

Paperback ISBN: 978-1-971996-57-8
Hardcover ISBN: 978-1-971996-58-5
E-book ISBN: 978-1-971996-59-2

Contents

Introduction

Fat loss is one of the most visible subjects in modern health culture, which is one reason it is so often misunderstood. It can be measured, photographed, compared, tracked, discussed, judged, and publicly displayed. A changing body or changing number appears concrete in a way many internal physiological processes do not. Because the visible outcome is easy to observe, the mechanism producing that outcome is often assumed to be equally simple.

This assumption creates distortion from the beginning.

When visible fat loss occurs, effort is often treated as the explanation. Restriction is credited. Exercise is credited. Discipline is credited. When visible change slows or reverses, the interpretation usually shifts toward personal failure. The person is assumed to have stopped trying, stopped caring, lost motivation, become inconsistent, or failed to maintain control. The visible outcome becomes moral evidence.

This book begins from a different position.

Fat loss is not denied here, minimized here, or dismissed as irrelevant. Stored reserves can decline. Body composition can change. Visible reduction can occur. But the purpose of this book is to explain that the visible outcome is not the mechanism itself. Fat loss is not simply effort converted into reduction. It is a regulated stored-energy outcome produced inside a larger metabolic system.

That distinction matters because visible outcomes can create the illusion that the body behaves like a direct-response machine. The assumption often looks simple: reduce intake, increase output, and stored energy should decline in a smooth and predictable way. There is truth inside that framework because stored reserves cannot decline without a relationship between incoming energy, outgoing energy, and stored energy. Energy balance matters. A body cannot continuously store more energy than it releases and simultaneously reduce reserves over long periods of time.

But energy balance is not self-executing.

The body does not experience reduced intake as arithmetic. It experiences reduced intake as a biological condition. Increased demand is interpreted biologically. Changing stored reserves are interpreted biologically. Stress, sleep disruption, appetite signaling, glucose behavior, movement demand, hormonal coordination, recovery capacity, and adaptation all influence how the system responds to changing energy conditions across time.

This means fat loss cannot be understood accurately through subtraction alone.

The body is not organized around producing visible reduction as its highest priority. The system is organized around continuity, survival, function, energy availability, repair, reproduction, movement, cognition, and long-horizon stability under changing environmental conditions. Stored energy exists inside that larger system.

For that reason, body fat is treated differently in this book than it often is in popular discussion. Stored energy is not framed here as moral failure, visual defect, or meaningless excess. It is reserve capacity. It is future availability. It participates in survival, stress buffering, recovery, hormonal signaling, and continuity across fluctuating conditions. That does not mean all levels of stored energy are metabolically neutral or physiologically identical. It means the system stores energy because storage serves a biological role.

Fat loss therefore requires more than simply wanting reduction to occur.

Stored energy first has to become accessible. The body regulates access according to feeding state, insulin tone, hormonal coordination, stress signaling, sleep quality, glycogen status, nervous system state, and demand conditions. Presence of stored energy alone does not guarantee that stored energy will meaningfully contribute to ongoing energy use.

Accessibility then has to continue into mobilization. Stored energy must move out of reserve form and into circulation. But even mobilization is not completion. Released energy can still return toward storage if it is not used strongly enough across time. Fat loss becomes meaningful only when stored energy continues through utilization. Tissues must require and use that energy within the broader energy environment of the body.

Storage and release therefore remain active together. The body does not enter a pure storage state or a pure release state permanently. Both processes continue interacting across time. Fat loss reflects the long-term direction of that balance rather than a simple on/off switch.

This immediately complicates the idea that fat loss is merely a direct output of discipline.

The system regulating stored energy is layered. Insulin participates in that regulation, but insulin is not treated in this book as a villain or singular master switch. It is a coordination signal involved in nutrient handling, fuel partitioning, uptake, storage conditions, and energy availability. Broader hormonal coordination also shapes the environment surrounding stored-energy use. Stress signaling, reproductive signaling, appetite signaling, thyroid-related regulation, sleep-related regulation, and nervous system state all influence the conditions under which stored energy is stored, accessed, released, or conserved.

No single variable controls the entire system.

Reduced energy availability also produces adaptation. When incoming energy remains lower relative to demand across time, the body may respond by narrowing the gap that originally supported visible loss. Output can decline. Efficiency can increase. Appetite pressure can rise.

Fatigue can increase. Recovery may become more difficult to maintain. The body is not necessarily malfunctioning when this occurs. It is adapting to a changing energy environment.

Compensation can emerge from those same conditions. Hunger may intensify. Food focus may increase. Cravings may become more prominent. Movement may decline without conscious intention. Task effort can feel more expensive. Fatigue can rise. These responses are often interpreted socially as weakness or loss of discipline, but the systems perspective is more precise: compensation reflects return pressure emerging under reduced energy availability and ongoing constraint.

This is one reason fat loss becomes difficult to interpret over time. The visible outcome is influenced by systems that continuously adjust underneath it.

Appetite becomes especially important in that environment because appetite is not simply preference. Hunger, cravings, satiety, food urgency, and food focus represent one behavioral interface of energy regulation. Appetite pressure can change when stored reserves decline, when intake changes, when glucose becomes unstable, when recovery deteriorates, when sleep worsens, when stress rises, or when compensation intensifies. The behavioral environment surrounding eating is therefore connected to internal regulation rather than existing separately from it.

Glucose behavior also matters, though not in the oversimplified way it is often discussed. Stable glucose does not guarantee fat loss, and unstable glucose does not make fat loss impossible. But glucose volatility can increase hunger, cravings, fatigue, urgency, and reactive eating pressure. It can destabilize perceived energy availability and increase compensation pressure around eating and output.

Demand matters as well. Released energy requires a destination. But demand should not be reduced to formal exercise alone. Daily movement, posture, task effort, work tolerance, fidgeting, spontaneous activity, training quality, recovery burden, and ordinary function all contribute to the broader energy environment. Output is not limited to workouts. Demand exists continuously across the day.

This also explains why visible progress is often inconsistent.

Plateaus can occur even when a person believes nothing has changed. But visible stalling does not automatically mean nothing is happening underneath. Water retention, glycogen shifts, digestive contents, recovery-related fluid changes, intake drift, stress load, adaptation, output reduction, and measurement variability can all influence visible weight and visible change. The scale is not a direct line into stored fat dynamics. It is a composite signal reflecting multiple interacting variables at once.

Rebound follows the same logic. Regain is often interpreted socially as proof that a person failed, lacked discipline, or stopped caring. This book approaches rebound differently. After fat loss occurs, the system may still carry appetite pressure, adaptation, lower output, environmental pull, stress burden, altered energy requirements, and old habit patterns. Return pressure can emerge if the new pattern has not stabilized strongly enough to hold against those combined forces.

None of this means fat loss is impossible.

It means fat loss is regulated.

That distinction changes how the process is interpreted. Instead of reducing outcomes to morality, motivation, or arithmetic alone, the systems model asks a different set of questions. Was stored energy accessible? Was mobilized energy consistently used? Did appetite pressure intensify? Did adaptation narrow the original gap? Did hidden output decline? Did stress or poor recovery increase compensation? Did rebound pressure emerge before stabilization occurred?

The goal of this book is not to provide a protocol that claims to overpower those variables. It is not a diet plan. It is not a calorie target system. It is not a fasting prescription. It is not an exercise manual. It is not a transformation narrative. It does not promise fat loss, and it does not treat visible reduction as proof of worth, discipline, or biological superiority.

It also does not frame fat mass, appetite, plateaus, or regain as moral evidence.

Instead, this book provides a systems model for understanding why fat loss can be inconsistent, why visible progress can slow, why appetite can intensify, why fatigue can rise, why plateaus occur, why rebound pressure appears, and why stable outcomes depend on coordination across time rather than force applied to a single variable.

The chapters that follow will examine stored energy, access, mobilization, utilization, insulin signaling, hormonal coordination, deficit signaling, adaptation, compensation, appetite pressure, glucose volatility, energy demand, plateaus, rebound pressure, and long-term stability as interacting parts of one system.

The purpose is not to simplify the process into one rule. The purpose is to make the process more interpretable.

Because fat loss is visible, it is often treated as though the visible outcome explains itself. This book argues the opposite. The visible outcome is the final surface expression of deeper regulatory processes operating underneath it. Those processes are dynamic, adaptive, compensatory, and context-dependent.

Fat loss therefore cannot be understood accurately as subtraction alone, and it cannot be understood accurately as personal virtue alone.

It must be understood as regulation across time.

Chapter 1 begins from that foundation by reframing fat loss itself not as a direct result of effort, but as a regulated system output produced inside a larger metabolic environment.

Fat Loss as a Regulated System Output

Fat loss often appears simpler than it is because the visible outcome seems easy to measure. Body weight changes. Clothing fit changes. Circumference changes. Food intake can be estimated. Activity can be tracked. The visible nature of these changes creates the impression that fat loss is a direct output of effort applied with enough consistency. A reduction in food intake appears as a controllable input. Increased movement appears as an adjustable variable. The resulting assumption is that stored body fat should respond in a relatively linear way when enough effort is sustained across time.

The simplicity of the visible outcome can obscure the complexity of the system producing it.

A change in stored energy is not generated by arithmetic alone. The body is not operating as a passive storage container waiting for instructions to remove energy. It is continuously coordinating energy availability, tissue demand, glucose regulation, appetite signaling, stress response, fluid balance, recovery needs, movement capacity, and functional continuity at the same time. Fat loss emerges from that coordinated environment rather than from intention alone.

This distinction matters because visible outcomes can create misleading interpretations of causation. When fat loss occurs, it is often interpreted as proof that effort directly caused the change. When fat loss slows or stops, the interruption is often interpreted as failure, inconsistency, lack of discipline, metabolic damage, or a broken system. Both interpretations compress a large regulatory process into a simple narrative of success or failure. The visible output becomes mistaken for the entire mechanism.

The body does not experience fat loss as a cosmetic event. It experiences changing energy conditions that must be interpreted and managed while preserving function. Stored energy exists inside a broader regulatory structure concerned with continuity, stability, and survival across time. A reduction in stored energy therefore depends not only on whether energy demand changes, but also on whether the system can continue operating while those changes occur.

This is one reason fat loss frequently becomes emotionally and conceptually entangled with effort. Effort is visible. Restriction is visible. Training is visible. The internal regulatory response is not. Appetite adjustments, stress accumulation, fatigue shifts, fluid retention, compensation, adaptive efficiency, and changes in spontaneous movement occur largely outside conscious observation. The hidden nature of these responses allows fat loss to appear more mechanically controllable than it actually is.

None of this means effort is irrelevant. Effort matters because changes in intake, activity, structure, and routine alter the conditions the system must regulate. But effort enters a biological environment that interprets those changes according to current energy availability, stress load, recovery status, hormonal signaling, and functional demand. The system responds to the total condition rather than to intention itself.

This creates an important distinction that will guide the rest of the book.

Effort is an input. Fat loss is an output. The relationship between them is mediated by regulation.

A person may reduce intake, increase movement, or apply more structure while assuming that stored energy reduction will occur in direct proportion to those actions. But the body is not responding only to reduced intake or increased demand. It is also adjusting hunger signals, movement efficiency, tissue repair priorities, glucose handling, fatigue perception, fluid balance, thermoregulation, and behavioral drive. These responses are not interruptions to the system. They are part of the system.

Because these adjustments occur simultaneously, the relationship between effort and fat loss is rarely perfectly linear. A person may believe the inputs are stable while underlying conditions continue shifting beneath the surface. Daily energy expenditure may decline slightly. Recovery demand may rise. Sleep disruption may alter appetite signaling. Increased stress may affect fluid retention and glucose variability. Reduced energy availability may influence movement outside deliberate exercise. The visible effort may remain consistent while the surrounding regulatory environment changes continuously.

This is where simplistic interpretations of fat loss often begin to fail. Linear models assume that the body responds to energy reduction with uncomplicated subtraction. Biological systems do not behave this way. They regulate, compensate, adapt, conserve, and prioritize simultaneously.

The existence of regulation does not invalidate energy balance. Stored energy cannot decrease without some relationship between incoming energy, outgoing energy, and stored reserves. Fat loss cannot occur independently of energy availability. The body cannot reduce stored tissue without a condition that permits stored energy utilization to exceed storage over time.

But energy balance is not self-executing.

The body does not experience a deficit as a spreadsheet instruction. It experiences changing energy availability as a series of biological signals. Reduced intake may alter hunger intensity, food focus, spontaneous movement, recovery capacity, or stress perception. Increased energy demand may affect fatigue, sleep quality, glucose stability, and tissue repair requirements. These responses influence whether the system continues permitting stored energy reduction under those conditions.

This distinction prevents two forms of oversimplification that commonly distort fat-loss discussions.

The first distortion treats calorie arithmetic as irrelevant. This interpretation suggests that stored energy changes occur independently of intake, expenditure, or availability. The second distortion treats calorie arithmetic as complete. This interpretation assumes that the body responds to changing energy conditions without adaptation, compensation, or regulation.

Neither position adequately describes how biological systems behave.

Energy balance matters because energy must come from somewhere. But the body regulates how energy is accessed, distributed, conserved, utilized, and defended while maintaining continuity across time. The existence of a deficit does not erase the system responsible for interpreting it.

This becomes especially important once fat loss extends beyond brief periods. The body is not merely reducing stored tissue in isolation. It is attempting to preserve function while energy conditions change.

Circulation must continue. Temperature regulation must continue. Glucose availability must remain sufficient for tissues that depend heavily on it. Cognitive function must continue. Tissue repair must continue. Daily movement must remain possible. Hormonal coordination must remain stable enough to preserve continuity across systems.

Fat loss therefore exists inside a larger negotiation between energy reduction and functional preservation.

If stored energy can be reduced while the system continues maintaining acceptable stability, fat loss may proceed with relatively manageable compensation. If energy reduction begins threatening functional continuity too aggressively, the system may increase protective responses. Appetite pressure may rise. Fatigue may increase. Recovery may become less efficient. Movement may unconsciously decline. Stress signaling may intensify. Water retention may shift. The body is not "refusing" fat loss in a conscious sense. It is regulating competing priorities simultaneously.

This is one reason rapid interpretations of stalled progress often become misleading. A slowdown in visible fat loss does not automatically mean that nothing is happening. Nor does it automatically mean the system is damaged. It may reflect shifting fluid balance, adaptive conservation, altered movement output, stress accumulation, recovery strain, or changes in stored glycogen. The visible output does not reveal the entire regulatory context beneath it.

The central issue is not whether fat loss can occur. It clearly can. The issue is whether stored energy reduction can continue without destabilizing function beyond what the system can tolerate for sustained continuity.

This chapter's governing mechanism emerges from that distinction.

Regulated Loss Mechanism: Fat loss occurs when stored energy can be reduced while the system preserves enough stability to continue functioning.

The mechanism contains two simultaneous conditions.

Stored energy must be reduced. Without a reduction in stored energy across time, fat loss does not occur.

At the same time, enough functional stability must remain intact for the system to continue operating without compensation escalating beyond sustainable continuity.

These two sides operate together. Fat loss cannot be understood accurately by isolating only one side of the equation. A model focused only on stored energy reduction ignores the regulatory burden placed on the system. A model focused only on preservation ignores the reality that fat loss requires actual reduction of stored reserves.

The interaction between these two conditions explains why fat loss can sometimes proceed relatively smoothly under one set of circumstances and become increasingly difficult under another, even when visible effort appears similar. The surrounding regulatory environment changes the system's interpretation of energy reduction.

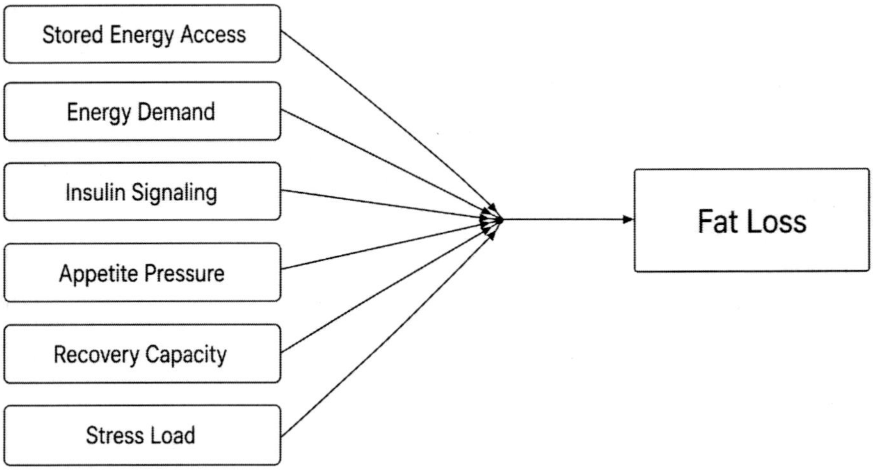

[Figure 1: Fat Loss as a Regulated Output]

The figure illustrates fat loss as a convergent output rather than a single lever. Stored energy access, energy demand, insulin signaling, appetite pressure, recovery capacity, and stress load all feed into the conditions under which fat loss occurs. No single variable independently determines the outcome. The body is coordinating multiple regulatory pressures simultaneously before stored energy reduction becomes visible as measurable fat loss.

This framing changes how inconsistency is interpreted.

Fat loss is often expected to behave in a smooth and predictable line because visible effort tends to be interpreted as the dominant causal factor. But visible consistency does not guarantee internal consistency. Many variables influencing stored energy behavior fluctuate beneath the surface even when routines appear unchanged.

Water retention can shift independently of fat mass. Glycogen storage changes with intake patterns, stress load, activity demand, and recovery state. Sleep disruption can alter appetite intensity and glucose behavior.

Psychological stress may influence fluid balance, recovery quality, and movement patterns. Hormonal signaling shifts continuously according to context. Daily movement outside structured exercise can rise or fall without deliberate awareness. Recovery strain may accumulate gradually across time rather than appearing immediately.

Adaptive efficiency also changes the equation. Systems exposed to repeated energy constraints may reduce unnecessary output, increase conservation, or alter behavioral drive in ways that influence total energy expenditure without conscious intention. These responses are not signs of malfunction. They are expressions of regulation.

Because these variables interact continuously, fat loss rarely behaves as a perfectly linear output even when a person believes the plan itself is unchanged. The visible result may temporarily accelerate, slow, stabilize, fluctuate, or reverse while multiple hidden variables reorganize simultaneously.

This nonlinearity often creates confusion because the visible signal is interpreted too narrowly. If scale weight changes are treated as the only meaningful indicator, short-term fluctuations may appear emotionally or biologically definitive. But body weight reflects more than stored fat alone. Water balance, glycogen status, digestive contents, inflammation, recovery demand, hormonal signaling, and stress exposure all influence the visible number at different times.

The body is not operating around the scale. The scale is observing one visible consequence of a much larger system.

This does not make measurement meaningless. It changes how measurement should be interpreted. A visible output becomes more useful when understood as part of a broader regulatory process rather than as a direct moral or mechanical verdict.

The same principle applies to effort itself. A person may interpret increased restriction or increased activity as proof that fat loss should accelerate proportionally. But greater intensity does not automatically improve system conditions. Under some circumstances, increased intensity may increase instability, recovery burden, appetite pressure, fatigue accumulation, or compensation faster than it improves stored energy reduction. The system experiences total stress load, not simply intended outcome.

This is one reason the book separates fat loss from transformation culture and performance framing. Transformation narratives often compress complex biological regulation into simplified stories of discipline, compliance, and visible reward. The body becomes portrayed as a machine that responds predictably when enough willpower is applied. But metabolic systems do not function independently of recovery capacity, hormonal coordination, glucose stability, appetite signaling, or adaptive protection.

Fat loss therefore cannot be understood accurately as a direct moral reward for effort. Nor can stalled fat loss be understood accurately as proof of personal failure. Both interpretations mistake visible output for complete explanation.

The purpose of this book is not to dismiss energy balance, deny physiology, or replace one simplistic model with another. Its purpose is to place fat loss back inside the regulatory environment that actually produces it.

Later chapters will examine how stored energy is mobilized, how energy access changes under different conditions, how insulin signaling influences storage and release dynamics, how appetite pressure interacts with energy availability, how adaptation alters expenditure and compensation, why plateaus emerge, why rebound occurs, and why maintenance conditions often determine whether fat loss remains stable across time.

Those mechanisms will matter because fat loss is not a standalone event. It is a sub-process occurring inside a larger metabolic system concerned with continuity.

This distinction changes the meaning of stability.

Fat loss stability is not the pursuit of the fastest possible reduction in stored energy. Faster loss does not automatically represent better regulation. The central question is whether the system can continue reducing stored energy without compensation escalating strongly enough to overwhelm continuity.

A system experiencing excessive compensation may produce increasing hunger, declining movement, impaired recovery, heightened fatigue, disrupted glucose regulation, greater stress load, or mounting instability that becomes progressively harder to sustain. In those conditions, fat loss may slow, stall, reverse, or become difficult to maintain once the surrounding structure changes.

The long-term problem is therefore not simply whether fat loss can be initiated. The problem is whether the conditions producing fat loss remain compatible with ongoing functional stability.

This book approaches fat loss through that lens.

It will not provide a transformation narrative, a motivational framework, or a prescriptive sequence promising guaranteed outcomes. It will not reduce body fat to a simple arithmetic contest between discipline and indulgence. It will not treat plateaus as proof of failure or adaptation as evidence that the system is broken.

Instead, it will examine how fat loss behaves when viewed as a regulated output produced by interacting conditions across time.

Fat loss begins under certain system conditions. It slows under others. It stalls, rebounds, accelerates, stabilizes, or destabilizes according to how the body interprets changing energy availability relative to recovery capacity, stress load, appetite pressure, hormonal signaling, and functional continuity.

The visible outcome matters, but the visible outcome is not the mechanism itself.

The mechanism is regulatory.

And fat loss stability ultimately depends on whether stored energy can be reduced without creating compensation strong enough to overwhelm the system's ability to continue functioning across time.

Fat Loss Is Not the Same as Weight Loss

Body weight is easy to notice because it produces a number. The number appears quickly, repeats easily, and seems objective. It can be compared across days, weeks, and months. Because of this visibility, body weight often becomes treated as if it directly explains fat change. When the number drops, fat loss is assumed. When the number rises, fat gain is assumed. When the number stalls, fat loss is assumed to have stopped.

The scale seems more explanatory than it is because it compresses several physical compartments into a single output.

A scale measures total body weight. It does not isolate fat mass. It does not distinguish stored energy from water, glycogen, digestive contents, sodium-related fluid shifts, inflammation, lean tissue, or temporary changes in food volume. The number is real, but its meaning is incomplete unless the compartments behind it are understood.

This distinction is foundational for fat loss stability. Fat loss refers to a slower change in stored energy. Weight loss refers to a reduction in total body weight, regardless of which compartment changed. These two processes can overlap, but they are not identical. A person can lose weight without losing much fat. A person can lose fat while total weight changes slowly. A person can experience a temporary increase in weight without reversing the longer process of stored-energy reduction.

The error is not measurement itself. The error is treating a composite signal as if it has only one cause.

Body weight is an aggregate. It is the combined mass of tissues, fluid, stored substrate, digestive material, and structural components. Fat mass is one part of that total, but it is not the only part that moves.

Water balance can change rapidly. Fluid shifts occur across compartments as the body adjusts circulation, sodium balance, tissue repair, temperature regulation, stress response, and hydration state. These changes can alter scale weight quickly without representing stored fat change.

Glycogen also influences weight because stored carbohydrate is held with water. When glycogen storage rises, associated water can increase total weight. When glycogen storage falls, associated water can decrease total weight. This can make the scale move visibly even when fat mass has not changed at the same speed.

Sodium-related fluid shifts can further alter body weight. Sodium helps regulate fluid distribution, and changes in sodium balance can influence how much water is retained or released. The resulting scale change may be noticeable, but it is not the same process as stored-energy reduction.

Inflammation and tissue repair can also affect fluid retention. When tissues are responding to stress, strain, or recovery demand, local and systemic fluid changes may occur. This can obscure changes in fat mass because the visible number reflects both stored-energy behavior and fluid regulation.

Digestive contents and food volume add another layer. Food and fluid moving through the digestive tract contribute temporary mass. This does not represent stored fat. It is part of total body weight at a given moment.

Lean tissue can change over longer periods as well. Muscle, connective tissue, organ mass, and other non-fat tissues are part of total body weight. These compartments do not fluctuate in the same way as water or digestive contents, but they remain part of the scale's total output.

Fat mass is different from these short-term compartments because it changes through stored-energy adjustment. It reflects the amount of energy held in adipose tissue and changes more slowly under ordinary conditions. Fat loss requires a sustained relationship between energy availability, stored energy access, and utilization across time. It does not rise and fall dramatically from one day to the next in the same way that fluid, glycogen, and digestive contents can.

This is why the scale can move quickly while fat mass moves slowly.

Fat loss is slower because it is not a temporary shift in content or fluid. It is a regulated change in stored energy. Stored fat must be accessed, mobilized, transported, and used within a broader system that is still maintaining glucose availability, appetite regulation, hormonal signaling, recovery, movement capacity, and daily function.

Water can shift quickly. Digestive contents can change within hours. Glycogen-associated water can change across short periods. Fat mass changes through a slower process because it reflects the cumulative reduction of stored energy, not the movement of temporary mass.

This explains several common patterns that are often misread.

Scale weight can drop quickly without much fat loss. In that case, the visible reduction may reflect fluid, glycogen, digestive contents, or food volume more than stored energy.

Scale weight can remain stable while fat loss may still be occurring. A slower reduction in fat mass can be masked by temporary increases in water retention, glycogen storage, digestive contents, or recovery-related fluid shifts.

Scale weight can rise temporarily while the longer-term fat trend has not reversed. A short-term increase does not automatically mean stored energy has increased. It may reflect a different compartment moving at the same time.

These patterns are not exceptions to the system. They are consequences of measuring a multi-compartment body with a single number.

Confusion between weight loss and fat loss creates false conclusions because it assigns single-cause meaning to a multi-cause signal.

Rapid early scale loss is often interpreted as rapid fat loss. Sometimes fat loss is part of the change, but the speed of the shift often reflects other compartments as well. Fluid, glycogen, food volume, and digestive contents can change faster than stored energy. When these rapid changes are mistaken for pure fat loss, expectations become distorted.

A temporary stall can be interpreted as failure. The assumption is that if the scale has not changed, fat loss must not be occurring. But a stable number may be the result of competing changes. Fat mass may be moving slowly while another compartment temporarily offsets the visible effect.

A short-term increase can be interpreted as regression. This interpretation assumes that weight gain and fat gain are identical. In reality, body weight may rise because of fluid, glycogen, sodium-related shifts, inflammation, digestive contents, or recovery demand. The number has changed, but the cause cannot be determined from the number alone.

The problem is not that body weight is useless. Body weight is one visible output of the system. The problem is over-reading it as a complete explanation. A single scale reading cannot identify which compartment changed. It can only report the combined result.

This distinction is especially important in fat loss because stored-energy change is often slower than the noise around it. Short-term volatility can hide the direction of the slower process. When the fast-moving compartments dominate attention, the slower regulated process becomes difficult to interpret.

The chapter's core mechanism is the Weight–Fat Separation Mechanism: body weight can change quickly across multiple compartments, while fat loss reflects slower stored-energy change.

This mechanism has two sides.

First, body weight is multi-compartment and responsive to short-term shifts. It can move because water changes, glycogen changes, sodium-related fluid shifts occur, digestive contents change, inflammation alters fluid retention, or lean tissue changes over time. The scale records the total of these movements without separating them.

Second, fat loss is a slower stored-energy process. It depends on the reduction of stored energy across time, not on every short-term movement in total mass.

Both sides must remain visible. If only the composite nature of body weight is emphasized, the scale may be dismissed completely. That would remove a potentially useful signal. If only stored-energy reduction is emphasized, scale volatility may continue to be over-interpreted as direct evidence of fat change.

The useful distinction is not that weight is false and fat is real. The useful distinction is that body weight is broad, while fat loss is specific.

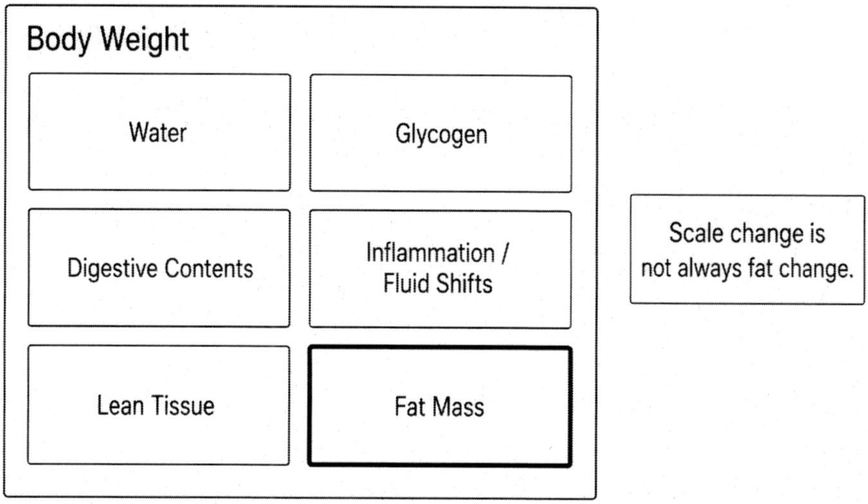

[Figure 2: Weight Change vs Fat Loss Compartments]

The figure shows body weight as a combined signal made up of several compartments. Water, glycogen, digestive contents, inflammation-related fluid shifts, lean tissue, and fat mass all contribute to the total. Fat mass is only one compartment within the larger measurement. This is why visible scale movement does not always reveal stored-energy change clearly.

The figure also clarifies why interpretation must be slower than measurement. The number may appear immediately, but the cause of the number requires context. A change in total body weight is not automatically a change in fat mass. It is a change in the combined output of all compartments contributing to body weight at that moment.

Measurement can still be useful because body weight is one visible output of the system. The issue is not the act of measuring. The issue is the meaning assigned to the measurement.

A single reading gives a momentary total. It does not explain composition, cause, direction, or mechanism. It does not reveal whether water moved, glycogen changed, digestive contents shifted, inflammation altered fluid retention, or fat mass changed. It provides a signal, not a full interpretation.

Body weight becomes more meaningful when understood as part of a broader pattern across time. This does not require turning measurement into an obsession or protocol. It simply means the number should be interpreted according to what it is: a total-body output influenced by multiple compartments.

This improves the frame for fat loss because it prevents the scale from being treated as a direct verdict on stored energy. It also prevents short-term volatility from overpowering the slower process that fat loss actually represents.

The body does not separate its compartments for the observer. The observer sees one number. The system underneath is managing fluid, substrate, tissue, digestion, recovery, and stored energy simultaneously.

Separating fat loss from weight loss is necessary for every mechanism that follows.

Stored energy access cannot be understood clearly if every scale drop is assumed to be fat loss. Mobilization cannot be understood clearly if temporary water shifts are mistaken for stored-energy change. Insulin signaling, appetite pressure, adaptation, plateaus, rebound, and maintenance all become distorted when total body weight is treated as a perfect stand-in for fat mass.

Fat loss is more specific than weight loss. It refers to the reduction of stored energy. Weight loss is broader. It may include fat mass, but it may also include water, glycogen, digestive contents, and other compartments. The two can occur together, but they do not always move together at the same speed or in the same direction.

This chapter does not reduce the value of body weight as information. It limits the conclusions that can be drawn from it. A visible number can be useful without being complete. A scale change can be real without being fully explanatory.

Fat loss stability depends on that interpretive separation. Without it, rapid changes are overvalued, stalls are misread, and short-term fluctuations are given more meaning than they can carry.

Fat loss is slower, more specific, and more regulated than scale volatility suggests.

Fat as Stored Energy, Not Excess

Body fat is often described as excess because it is visible, measurable, and culturally interpreted long before it is biologically explained. The language surrounding fat mass frequently assumes that stored energy exists primarily as a problem to be corrected or removed. Terms such as excess weight or excess fat appear neutral at first glance, but they already contain an interpretation. They imply that the stored tissue has little functional significance beyond representing more than what should be present.

From a systems perspective, this framing creates distortion before the mechanism is even examined.

"Excess" is not a neutral biological category. It is a judgment layered onto a storage system. It compresses multiple functions into a simplified conclusion that the tissue exists only as surplus material. Once this assumption becomes dominant, fat loss is interpreted primarily as disposal rather than as a regulated change within a broader metabolic environment.

This chapter begins from a different position. Before body fat can be interpreted, it must first be defined according to function.

The body stores energy because biological systems operate across changing conditions. Incoming energy is not always synchronized perfectly with outgoing demand. Activity changes. Recovery demand changes. Food availability changes. Stress exposure changes. Sleep quality changes. Illness, injury, workload, seasonality, schedule disruption, and fasting intervals all alter the relationship between energy intake and energy use. A system dependent entirely on immediate intake would become fragile whenever conditions shifted.

Stored energy reduces that fragility.

Fat mass represents one of the body's primary methods of preserving future energy availability across time. Energy consumed during one period can remain accessible during another period when intake decreases, demand rises, or conditions become less predictable. This is not a design error within the system. It is part of how long-horizon continuity is maintained.

Seen through this lens, fat tissue is not merely accumulation. It is reserve capacity.

This does not mean that all levels of fat storage are physiologically equivalent or that variation in fat mass carries no metabolic consequences. The point is narrower and more foundational. Before fat loss can be understood clearly, body fat must first be understood as a regulated energy compartment rather than as symbolic evidence of failure, discipline, control, or worth.

The body does not store energy randomly. Storage occurs because future conditions cannot be predicted with perfect precision in advance. Systems operating across uncertain environments require mechanisms that bridge the gap between present availability and future demand. Stored energy provides that bridge.

The importance of this distinction becomes clearer when energy regulation is viewed across time instead of only within isolated moments. Food intake happens episodically. Energy demand is continuous. The body therefore requires methods for maintaining continuity between periods of intake and periods of use. Some of this continuity is managed through circulating nutrients and short-term storage systems, but longer-term reserve capacity is also necessary.

Fat mass serves that longer-horizon reserve function.

A person may consume energy during one portion of the day while requiring energy hours later during movement, cognition, tissue repair, thermoregulation, immune activity, or basic physiological maintenance. Over longer periods, demand may rise while intake falls. Sleep disruption may alter energy regulation. Illness may increase recovery needs. Psychological stress may influence intake patterns and output simultaneously. The metabolic system therefore operates under conditions where immediate balance is constantly shifting.

Stored energy helps stabilize those shifts.

This is why fat storage is more accurately understood as a buffer than as passive excess.

In systems terms, a buffer reduces fragility when inputs fluctuate. It creates reserve capacity that allows the system to continue functioning despite variation in conditions. Mechanical systems use buffers to absorb pressure variation. Financial systems use reserves to maintain continuity during instability. Biological systems also rely on reserve structures because living systems operate in environments that are dynamic rather than fixed.

Metabolically, stored energy functions as one of those reserve structures.

Without reserve capacity, every reduction in intake would immediately threaten continuity. Every increase in demand would create greater instability. The body would remain dependent on constant real-time replenishment without a mechanism for bridging variability across time.

Fat storage helps prevent that kind of immediate fragility.

This does not mean the system seeks unlimited storage or that all storage patterns are equally adaptive under all conditions. Buffers themselves require regulation. Too little reserve capacity increases vulnerability to instability. Excessive storage under certain conditions may alter signaling, mobility, energy regulation, or metabolic coordination. But those later questions cannot be interpreted accurately if fat tissue is first reduced to meaningless accumulation.

The existence of stored energy reflects a functional principle before it becomes a cultural interpretation.

This framing also changes how fat loss itself is understood. If fat tissue represents stored energy with reserve value, then fat loss is not merely subtraction. It is a change in a reserve system the body may attempt to regulate according to current and anticipated conditions.

The body does not treat stored energy as inert material with no future importance. Stored energy has regulatory value because it represents future availability. As a result, conditions influencing perceived stability can influence how the system responds to stored reserves.

When energy availability appears unstable, protective pressure may increase. When stress load rises, the system may respond as if future demands are becoming less predictable. When recovery becomes inadequate, compensatory responses may increase. When signaling becomes inconsistent, the body may regulate energy storage and release differently than it would under more stable conditions.

These responses do not require conscious intention. The body is not making psychological decisions about fat mass. Regulation emerges from coordinated signaling, feedback loops, substrate availability, hormonal communication, and adaptive pressure across systems.

The important distinction is that stored energy is not metabolically silent.

Conditions can increase or decrease pressure toward storage, maintenance, or release depending on how the system interprets the broader environment. This interpretation occurs physiologically through signals related to energy availability, stress exposure, recovery status, glucose behavior, hormonal coordination, and ongoing demand.

This is one reason fat loss cannot be understood purely through visible mass alone. The stored-energy compartment participates in broader regulation. Changes in stored energy influence signaling environments rather than existing independently from them.

Fat tissue is therefore more than a storage depot.

It participates in communication.

Fat mass interacts with hormonal signaling related to energy status, appetite regulation, and broader metabolic coordination. The body uses information about stored energy availability as part of how it regulates intake pressure, expenditure behavior, and longer-term stability. This does not mean fat tissue controls the entire system independently, nor does it mean every change in fat mass produces simple or predictable outcomes. The point is more restrained: stored energy communicates information about energy conditions.

Fat mass is storage, but it is not silent storage.

This matters because regulatory systems behave differently when reserve capacity changes. A reduction in stored energy is not interpreted only as a change in appearance or total mass. It may also alter the signaling environment connected to energy availability and future reserve status.

The body therefore regulates fat tissue according to more than immediate arithmetic. Current intake matters. Current expenditure matters. But the surrounding environment also matters because stored energy functions inside a larger system attempting to maintain continuity across time.

This chapter's central mechanism emerges from that relationship.

The Stored Energy Buffer Mechanism describes body fat as an energy reserve that the system protects, releases, or maintains depending on perceived conditions.

Three broad regulatory patterns can emerge from this mechanism.

Under conditions associated with instability, scarcity, or strain, protective pressure may increase. When energy availability appears uncertain, when recovery capacity narrows, or when stress signaling intensifies, the body may regulate stored energy more conservatively. This does not mean fat loss becomes impossible. It means the system may behave as if preserving reserve capacity has become more important.

Under conditions where access and demand are aligned appropriately, stored energy may be released and utilized more effectively. In these situations, reserve capacity becomes available for ongoing energy use without destabilizing broader function excessively.

Under relatively stable conditions, the system may also tend toward maintenance. When current patterns appear sufficiently matched to ongoing demand, stored energy may remain relatively stable rather than shifting dramatically toward either rapid accumulation or rapid release.

These are not behavioral instructions or fixed categories. They are regulatory tendencies reflecting how reserve systems operate under changing conditions.

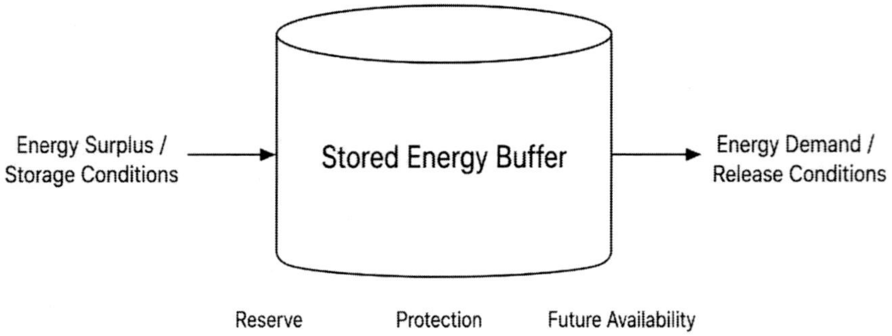

[Figure 3: Fat as Stored Energy Buffer]

The figure presents body fat as a reserve positioned between storage conditions and release conditions. Incoming energy surplus and storage-supportive conditions feed into the stored-energy buffer, while energy demand and release-supportive conditions draw from it. The buffer itself represents reserve capacity rather than passive accumulation. Stored energy can be filled, maintained, protected, or utilized depending on the broader state of the system.

The figure also clarifies that fat storage is not isolated from context. Storage and release do not occur independently from signaling conditions, recovery state, stress exposure, or ongoing energy demand. The stored-energy compartment exists within a dynamic regulatory environment rather than functioning as a static container.

This becomes especially important once fat loss itself is examined more closely.

If body fat is interpreted only as unwanted excess, fat loss appears conceptually simple. The existence of stored energy seems to imply immediate availability for removal. But if stored energy has reserve value, signaling roles, and continuity functions, then fat loss becomes more than disposal. It becomes the reduction of a regulated reserve compartment.

That distinction changes the questions the rest of the book must answer.

The central issue is no longer simply whether stored energy exists. The issue becomes whether stored energy is accessible under current conditions, how the body regulates that access, what signals increase protective pressure, what conditions support release and utilization, and how compensation emerges when stability begins narrowing.

The existence of stored energy does not automatically guarantee access to stored energy.

A reservoir can exist while access remains restricted. A reserve can be present while the system simultaneously increases appetite pressure, conserves expenditure, alters movement patterns, or adjusts signaling in ways that complicate release. The body is not merely responding to the quantity of stored energy. It is responding to the broader environment surrounding that stored energy.

This is why fat loss cannot be reduced accurately to a simple removal model. Stored energy exists within a regulatory system concerned with continuity, not only with reduction.

The misunderstanding created by the word "excess" becomes clearer here. If fat tissue is treated as biologically meaningless, any resistance to rapid reduction appears irrational or pathological. But if fat tissue functions as reserve capacity, then regulatory protection becomes more understandable. The body is not responding only to present conditions. It is regulating future availability under uncertainty.

Again, this does not imply conscious planning by the system. It reflects the behavior of adaptive regulatory mechanisms shaped around continuity across fluctuating environments.

This perspective also prevents the opposite oversimplification. Explaining fat tissue as functional reserve does not mean every storage pattern is metabolically neutral under all circumstances or that unlimited storage carries no physiological consequences. The purpose of this chapter is not to idealize fat accumulation. It is to explain why the compartment exists and why regulation surrounds it.

A reserve system cannot be understood clearly if its reserve function is ignored.

The broader argument of this book depends on that foundation. Later chapters will examine stored-energy access, mobilization, utilization, insulin signaling, adaptation, compensation, plateaus, and rebound. Each of those processes assumes that body fat is operating as regulated stored energy rather than as passive excess waiting to disappear.

Chapter 2 separated fat loss from weight loss by clarifying that body weight is a composite signal. This chapter defines the specific compartment underneath that distinction. Fat mass represents stored energy maintained within a regulatory environment shaped by future availability, stability demands, and adaptive signaling.

The next question therefore becomes unavoidable.

If fat tissue is stored energy, under what conditions is that stored energy actually available for use?

That question leads directly into the next chapter because the presence of stored energy and the accessibility of stored energy are not identical conditions.

Fat loss depends not only on how much stored energy exists, but also on the regulatory conditions that allow the system to release and utilize it without destabilizing continuity beyond what it can sustain.

Fat loss therefore begins with a more accurate definition of fat itself.

Not excess to be eliminated.

Stored energy governed by regulation.

Stored Energy Is Not Always Accessible

If body fat is stored energy and reserve capacity, the next question is not simply how much stored energy exists. The next question is whether that stored energy is available for use.

A reserve can be present without being open. Stored energy can exist without being actively drawn upon. This distinction is central to fat loss because the presence of fat mass does not automatically mean the system is using that stored energy in a meaningful way. The body does not treat reserve energy as a constantly open fuel source. It regulates access according to current conditions.

This does not mean stored energy is unreachable or permanently protected. It means access is conditional. Biological reserves are not passive piles of material waiting to be removed. They are regulated compartments shaped by signaling, demand, availability, and stability. The system may protect stored energy under one set of conditions, maintain it under another, and release it under another.

Chapter 3 defined fat as stored energy rather than excess. That framing matters here because stored energy has reserve value. A reserve with future value is not released without regulation. The body tends to coordinate access according to whether current conditions support release, circulation, and use while preserving broader function.

Stored energy and available energy are therefore not the same condition.

Stored energy is energy held in reserve. It exists as capacity for future use. Available energy is energy that can enter circulation and contribute to current demand. Fat loss depends on movement from storage toward availability, but that movement is not automatic. The reserve must become accessible before it can meaningfully contribute to ongoing energy use.

This is where simplistic fat-loss thinking often breaks down. If stored energy is present, it can seem logical to assume that reduced intake or increased demand should immediately force the body to use it. But the body does not operate by direct command. It interprets changing intake, output, stress, recovery, glucose behavior, and hormonal signals as part of one regulatory environment.

Access is the checkpoint between storage and use.

Stored fat must move out of reserve status before it can enter the usable energy stream. That transition involves release, circulation, and eventual use by tissues. The presence of stored fat alone does not complete that sequence. It only establishes that reserve energy exists.

The system must also permit movement from storage toward availability.

This checkpoint is influenced by several overlapping conditions. None of them acts as a single switch. They operate together, shaping whether stored energy is more protected, more available, or relatively unchanged under the current state of the system.

Insulin tone is one of the major signals influencing this access point. Insulin is not a moral signal, a failure signal, or an enemy of fat loss. It is a coordination signal. It helps the body interpret incoming energy, distribute nutrients, support storage, and regulate release. When insulin tone is higher, the system generally favors nutrient storage and reduced release from stored reserves. When insulin tone is lower, stored energy access may become more permissive, depending on the broader state of the system.

This does not make insulin the only variable. It also does not mean lower insulin tone automatically produces fat loss. Access still depends on total energy availability, demand, stress state, recovery, and hormonal coordination. Insulin participates in the access environment; it does not replace the entire system.

Recent feeding also influences access because incoming energy changes priority. After food intake, the system often gives attention to absorbed nutrients entering circulation. Energy is arriving from outside the reserve. Under those conditions, reliance on stored reserves may be reduced because incoming energy is available to meet current needs, refill shorter-term stores, and support ongoing function.

This is not a rule about meal timing. It is a systems observation. When usable energy is entering the system, stored energy may become less immediately necessary. When incoming energy is lower or absent, stored reserves may become more relevant, but only if other access conditions support release and use.

Glycogen status adds another layer. Glycogen functions as a shorter-term energy reserve, especially relevant to glucose availability and activity demand. When glycogen availability is higher, the system may rely more readily on that shorter-term reserve for certain demands. When glycogen availability declines, reliance on stored fat may increase under some conditions. But this relationship should not be flattened into a single dietary argument. Glycogen is one part of the access environment, not the whole explanation.

Stored fat exists in a hierarchy of energy availability. Some energy is immediate. Some is short-term. Some is longer-term. The body coordinates across these layers rather than drawing from all reserves equally at all times.

Stress state also influences access, though not in the simplistic sense that stress simply blocks fat loss. Stress alters the regulatory environment. It can affect glucose availability, counter-regulatory signaling, appetite pressure, fluid balance, sleep quality, recovery demand, and perceived energy need. Under certain conditions, stress may increase reliance on glucose availability or increase compensatory pressure that changes how stored energy is accessed and used.

The important point is not that stress makes fat loss impossible. It is that stress changes the context in which energy access is regulated. A system under higher strain may interpret reduced intake or increased demand differently from a system operating with more stable recovery and coordination.

Sleep and recovery shape the same access environment. Recovery is not separate from metabolism. It supports signal clarity, tissue repair, hormonal rhythm, appetite regulation, glucose handling, and energy continuity. When recovery is insufficient, the system may face greater compensatory pressure. Fatigue may rise. Appetite signals may intensify. Movement output may decline. Glucose behavior may become less stable. These changes can alter the conditions under which stored energy is accessed.

Access requires coordination. Recovery supports coordination. When recovery capacity narrows, the system may still access stored energy, but the process may occur with more friction, compensation, or instability.

Activity demand also matters because stored energy becomes more relevant when tissues require energy. Demand creates a reason for fuel to be made available. Movement, tissue repair, thermoregulation, and daily function all require energy. Stored reserves become meaningful when current demand exceeds what is immediately available from incoming or circulating sources.

But more demand is not automatically better. Demand enters the same regulatory environment as every other signal. If activity demand rises beyond recovery capacity, the system may respond with fatigue, conservation, appetite pressure, or stress signaling. The useful distinction is that demand can increase the relevance of stored energy, but demand must still be integrated with stability.

Hormonal coordination gives this process its broader structure. Stored energy access is not governed by one hormone acting alone. Insulin, counter-regulatory signals, appetite-related signals, stress-related signals, and tissue-level feedback all interact to regulate availability and use. The system does not operate as one switch flipped from storage to release. It operates as coordinated signal interpretation across time.

Broader energy availability ties these conditions together. The body regulates access according to the total environment: incoming energy, stored reserves, current demand, recovery state, stress load, glucose stability, hormonal signaling, and perceived continuity. Access becomes easier to understand when it is viewed as a system decision rather than a single biochemical event.

The Stored Energy Access Mechanism defines this chapter's central claim: fat loss requires stored energy to become available, not merely present.

The mechanism has two parts.

The first is presence. Stored energy exists as reserve capacity. Fat mass is present in the body as stored energy that may be used under certain conditions.

The second is access. Stored energy becomes available for release, circulation, and use. Without access, stored energy remains a reserve rather than a current contributor to energy demand.

Fat loss is constrained when presence exists without access. This is why the amount of stored energy alone does not determine the ease, speed, or stability of fat loss. A body may have stored energy present while the system still regulates availability conservatively under certain conditions. The reserve exists, but the access point is constrained.

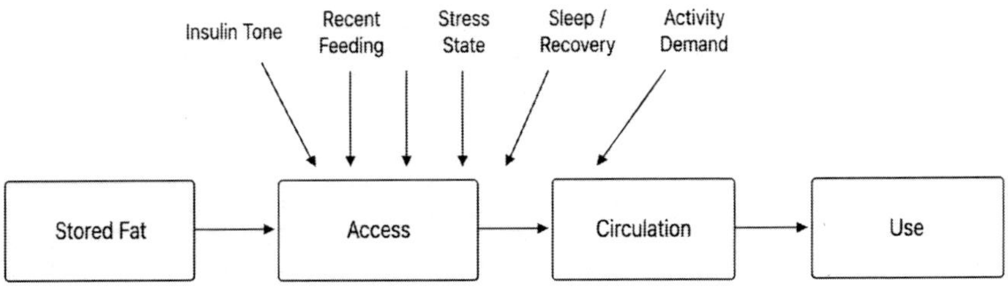

[Figure 4: Stored Fat → Access → Circulation → Use]

The figure shows access as the transition point between stored energy and usable energy. Stored fat must move through an access stage before it can enter circulation and be used by tissues. The labels above the access point—insulin tone, recent feeding, stress state, sleep and recovery, and activity demand—show that this step is influenced by multiple conditions rather than controlled by intention alone.

The figure also clarifies sequence. Stored fat is not the same as energy already being used. Access precedes circulation. Circulation precedes use. Use must occur before stored energy reduction becomes meaningful as fat loss. The system can be interrupted, slowed, or constrained at different points in that sequence.

This distinction matters because many fat-loss interpretations assume that stored energy should be immediately available whenever intake decreases. When that does not happen smoothly, the result is often interpreted as failure, broken metabolism, or lack of effort. A systems view provides a more precise explanation. Stored energy may be present, while current conditions make access less efficient, more restricted, or more costly.

This can create the paradox that confuses many interpretations of fat loss: stored reserves may exist while the person experiences fatigue, hunger, reduced output, or compensation. From a simple storage model, this seems illogical. If energy exists, why would the system behave as if energy is limited? From a regulatory model, the answer is clearer. Energy that is stored is not the same as energy that is available.

Fatigue can appear when the system does not readily move stored energy into usable circulation at the rate current demand requires. Hunger can increase when the body interprets incoming energy or available energy as insufficient. Compensation can rise when energy reduction, stress load, and recovery demand begin narrowing functional stability. Reduced output can occur when the system conserves energy rather than expanding access smoothly.

These are not necessarily signs of pathology. They are expressions of regulation under constraint.

The same principle explains why fat loss can feel inconsistent even when effort appears stable. The amount of stored energy may not be the limiting factor. Access conditions may shift. Insulin tone may change with recent intake and rhythm. Stress may alter glucose handling and fluid balance. Sleep may affect appetite and recovery. Activity demand may increase faster than recovery capacity. Hormonal signals may become less coordinated. The reserve remains present, but the pathway from reserve to usable energy changes.

This is why Chapter 4 sits at the center of the book's foundation. Before mobilization can be discussed, access must be understood. Before release can be interpreted, the system must permit stored energy to move out of reserve status. Before utilization can be evaluated, the energy must become available to tissues.

Fat loss requires a sequence, not merely a stored compartment.

Stored energy must become accessible. Accessible energy must be released. Released energy must circulate. Circulating energy must be used.

The process is regulated at each stage by conditions that influence whether the system can reduce stored energy while preserving function.

The next chapter moves into mobilization. Once stored energy becomes accessible, it may be released from storage. But release is not the same as fat loss. Mobilization creates movement from the reserve, but permanent reduction depends on what happens afterward.

Stored energy must become accessible before it can be released, circulated, and used. That access point is where the reserve begins to shift from stored capacity toward usable energy.

Mobilization Is Not the Same as Fat Loss

Chapter 4 established that stored energy must become accessible before it can contribute to usable energy. The existence of stored fat alone does not guarantee that the system is actively drawing from it. Access represents the transition point between reserve capacity and availability. Once that transition occurs, another stage begins: mobilization.

Mobilization means stored fat has moved out of storage into a more available state. Energy that was previously held in reserve becomes released into circulation where it may contribute to current demand. This movement is necessary for fat loss because stored energy cannot be reduced without first leaving storage.

But mobilization should not be mistaken for completion.

The release of stored fat is not the same as permanent reduction of stored fat. Movement out of storage begins the process, but it does not finish it. Released energy must still follow a path that leads toward sustained use. Without that continuation, mobilized energy may remain temporary, circulate briefly, or return toward storage rather than producing meaningful long-term reduction in stored reserves.

This distinction matters because fat loss is often described too simplistically. Once stored fat is released, the process is frequently treated as complete. Common "fat-burning" language reinforces this assumption by collapsing multiple stages into one event. But the body does not treat release and loss as identical conditions. Stored energy can move out of reserve status without producing durable reduction if the broader system environment does not support continued use.

Mobilization therefore represents movement from storage toward use, not guaranteed loss by itself.

This is easier to understand when release and reduction are separated conceptually.

Release describes movement out of storage. Stored energy becomes mobilized and enters a more available state. Reduction describes a sustained decrease in the stored reserve itself. Reduction occurs when released energy is ultimately used over time in a way that lowers the amount remaining in storage.

The difference between these two stages explains why mobilization alone cannot define fat loss. A reserve can be opened temporarily without meaningfully shrinking across time. Energy can leave storage briefly and still return if conditions support re-storage more strongly than sustained use.

This does not make mobilization irrelevant. Mobilization is essential. Stored fat cannot contribute to energy use without first leaving storage. But the presence of mobilization only confirms that movement has begun. It does not confirm where the released energy ultimately goes.

Once mobilized, fatty acids can follow several possible paths.

They can be used by tissues that require energy. They can remain circulating temporarily while the system determines demand and substrate preference. Or they can return toward storage if competing conditions make continued use less likely or less necessary.

The broader metabolic environment influences which direction becomes more dominant.

Energy demand is one of the most important factors shaping the post-mobilization pathway. Released energy becomes more relevant when tissues require fuel. Movement, thermoregulation, tissue repair, organ function, and daily activity all create ongoing demand for usable energy.

Mobilized fatty acids are more likely to contribute to reduction when the system continues directing them toward active use.

Demand creates a destination for released fuel.

Without sufficient demand, released energy may remain temporarily available without being meaningfully utilized. The body regulates energy continuously, and fuel entering circulation does not automatically disappear from the system simply because it left storage. It must still contribute to ongoing energy requirements strongly enough and consistently enough to reduce the reserve over time.

Competing fuel availability also influences this process. The body often has access to multiple potential fuel sources simultaneously. Incoming nutrients, circulating glucose, glycogen reserves, and mobilized fatty acids all exist within the broader energy environment. When incoming or circulating energy is already available in sufficient quantity, mobilized fatty acids may not be prioritized for sustained use.

This does not mean mobilization failed. It means release occurred within an environment where alternative fuel availability altered what happened afterward.

The system coordinates among available fuels rather than treating mobilized fat as automatically dominant once released. If incoming energy continues meeting demand effectively, released fatty acids may circulate temporarily or return toward storage instead of contributing to meaningful reduction of the reserve.

Insulin signaling remains part of this post-release environment as well. Insulin continues influencing how energy is directed, distributed, stored, or utilized. Higher insulin tone generally supports storage-related processes and may reduce the likelihood that mobilized fatty acids continue moving toward sustained use. Lower insulin tone may permit greater reliance on mobilized energy under some conditions, but insulin is still only one component within a larger regulatory system.

The system does not decide energy direction based on insulin alone. Demand, recovery state, substrate availability, stress load, and broader coordination remain involved throughout the process. Insulin participates in shaping the post-mobilization environment rather than functioning as a solitary controller of fat loss.

Activity state further influences whether mobilized energy becomes meaningful reduction. Tissues requiring energy create conditions where circulating fuel becomes more relevant. Movement increases energy turnover, and mobilized fatty acids may contribute more directly to current demand when energy requirements rise appropriately.

But activity should not be interpreted as a simple prescription or a direct guarantee of fat loss. More activity is not automatically better if it simultaneously increases stress load, recovery strain, or compensatory pressure faster than the system can stabilize. The body responds to total demand within the broader context of recovery capacity and system coordination.

Mobilization becomes more useful when demand and recovery remain sufficiently aligned for released energy to continue moving toward use rather than cycling back toward storage.

Metabolic flexibility also shapes this process. The body continuously shifts among available fuel sources according to changing conditions. A system with greater flexibility can transition between glucose use, glycogen use, and fat-derived energy more effectively as availability and demand change. This flexibility influences whether mobilized fatty acids can continue moving toward utilization once released.

If the system struggles to transition efficiently between substrates under certain conditions, released energy may not be directed toward sustained use as effectively. Mobilization can still occur, but continued contribution to energy demand may become less stable or less coordinated.

This is one reason fat loss cannot be understood only through the moment of release. The broader ability of the system to integrate and utilize changing fuel availability matters as much as the existence of mobilization itself.

Stress load also alters the post-mobilization environment. Stress changes glucose behavior, substrate preference, hormonal coordination, appetite signaling, and recovery demand. Under some conditions, stress may increase reliance on more rapidly available energy sources or alter how efficiently mobilized fatty acids are directed toward sustained use.

Again, this should not be simplified into claims that stress "prevents" fat loss. The more accurate explanation is that stress changes the context in which mobilized energy is processed. Higher stress load may increase compensatory pressure, alter recovery quality, influence appetite behavior, and narrow stability margins. These changes affect what happens after release occurs.

Recovery state operates alongside stress in the same broader environment. Mobilization becomes more meaningful when the system can sustain coordinated use without excessive compensation. Poor recovery may increase fatigue, reduce spontaneous movement, destabilize appetite signals, impair sleep quality further, or narrow the body's tolerance for continued energy reduction.

Released energy exists within this recovery context rather than outside it.

The same mobilization event may produce different outcomes under different recovery conditions because the body is regulating more than fuel movement alone. It is also preserving continuity across cognition, tissue repair, immune function, hormonal rhythm, and daily capacity.

System stability ultimately ties these variables together. Mobilization contributes most effectively to fat loss when release, demand, signaling, recovery, and fuel use remain sufficiently coordinated across time. When these conditions align, released energy is more likely to continue moving toward utilization rather than cycling temporarily through circulation and returning toward storage.

This chapter's governing mechanism emerges from that distinction.

The Mobilization Constraint Mechanism states that stored fat must be released under conditions that allow continued use rather than simple cycling or re-storage.

The mechanism has two connected parts.

The first part is release from storage. Stored fat becomes mobilized and enters a more available state. This represents movement out of reserve status and into circulation.

The second part is post-release direction. Once mobilized, energy may move toward sustained use, remain circulating temporarily, or return toward storage depending on the broader state of the system.

The central constraint is therefore not whether mobilization can occur at all. Mobilization occurs regularly within normal metabolic regulation. The more important question is whether the conditions surrounding mobilization support continued use strongly enough to reduce the reserve across time.

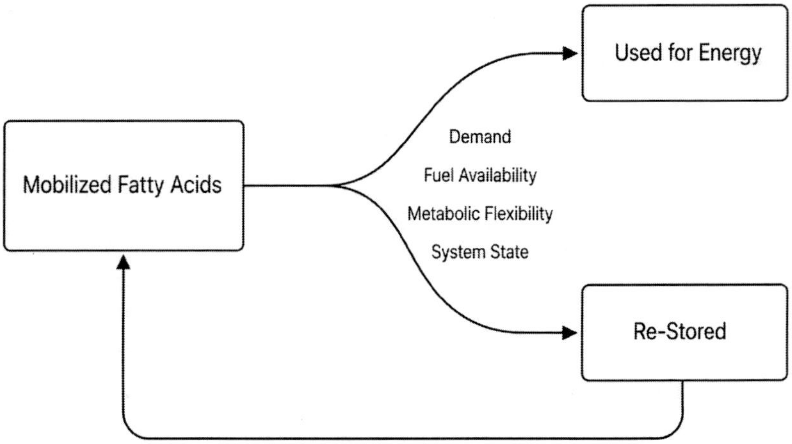

[Figure 5: Mobilized Fat: Used vs Re-Stored]

The figure presents mobilized fat at a branch point rather than as a completed outcome. Once stored energy is released, it can move toward use or return toward storage depending on conditions such as energy demand, fuel availability, metabolic flexibility, and broader system state. The diagram prevents release from being mistaken for permanent loss. Mobilization begins movement away from storage, but the path after release remains regulated.

The figure also illustrates why "fat-burning" language can become misleading when interpreted too literally. A temporary increase in mobilization does not automatically mean that stored reserves are declining meaningfully across time. Released energy may circulate briefly without producing sustained reduction if competing conditions favor re-storage or reduce ongoing use.

This distinction helps explain why short-term interpretations of fat loss often become distorted. A person may experience periods where mobilization increases transiently without seeing a large visible change in stored reserves. From a simplistic perspective, this can appear contradictory. If fat was released, why did meaningful reduction not occur?

The systems explanation is more precise. Release alone does not determine outcome. Mobilized energy still requires continued direction toward use.

This is also why the body cannot be understood as operating through isolated events. Mobilization is one stage in a larger sequence. Access precedes mobilization. Utilization follows mobilization. Fat loss becomes meaningful when these stages continue coherently enough to reduce reserve capacity across time.

The broader environment surrounding mobilization determines whether the process continues or loops backward.

A system experiencing high competing fuel availability may mobilize energy while simultaneously reducing the need for continued use of that energy. A system under high stress load may alter substrate preference or compensation patterns after release occurs. A system with insufficient recovery may mobilize energy while also reducing movement output, increasing fatigue, or intensifying appetite pressure in ways that complicate sustained reduction.

None of these outcomes make mobilization irrelevant. They clarify its position within the overall pathway.

Fat loss requires coordination across stages rather than isolated activation of one mechanism.

This perspective also reframes how short-term "fat-burning" claims are often interpreted in broader health culture. Temporary increases in mobilization are frequently treated as proof that meaningful fat loss is occurring immediately. But release from storage and durable reduction of stored reserves are not identical conditions. The body may increase mobilization transiently while the longer-term storage balance remains relatively stable.

This is why the book separates mobilization from utilization rather than collapsing them into one event.

Mobilization is necessary because stored energy cannot be used while remaining locked in reserve status. But release alone does not complete the process. The system must continue directing that released energy toward ongoing use strongly enough and consistently enough for stored reserves to decline across time.

The next chapter therefore moves to utilization itself.

Once stored energy has become accessible and mobilized, the remaining question is whether tissues actually use that energy in a sustained way. Circulating fuel must become functional energy expenditure before mobilization becomes meaningful fat loss.

Fat loss requires more than release.

It requires a coordinated path from release toward continued use.

Utilization: Released Energy Must Be Used

Mobilization begins the movement of stored energy out of reserve status, but it does not complete fat loss by itself. Chapter 5 separated release from reduction by showing that stored fat can be mobilized without necessarily producing durable change in the stored reserve. Once energy has left storage and entered a more available state, the next question becomes whether that released energy is actually used.

This is the final stage of the first major pathway in fat loss: stored energy must become accessible, then mobilized, then utilized.

Utilization is the point where released fuel becomes functional energy use. It is not simply the presence of fatty acids in circulation or the fact that stored energy has left its original compartment. It is the use of that energy by tissues to support work, maintenance, repair, movement, thermoregulation, cognition, immune activity, and the continuous operations of daily physiology.

Mobilization creates possibility. Utilization creates functional consequence.

This distinction matters because fuel released from storage does not automatically disappear from the body. It does not become meaningful fat loss merely because it has entered circulation. Released energy requires a destination. It must be taken up and used by tissues in a sustained enough pattern to contribute to reduction of the stored reserve over time.

If released energy is not used strongly enough or consistently enough, the result may be temporary circulation, displacement by other fuels, or eventual return toward storage. The reserve may have opened, but the reduction may not become durable.

The body is constantly coordinating fuel movement with fuel demand. Energy does not become useful simply because it is available. It becomes useful when a tissue requires it, can take it up, and can process it into functional output. This is why utilization must be separated from mobilization. Mobilization moves energy into a more available state. Utilization determines whether that availability becomes actual use.

Demand is the central reason released energy becomes relevant.

Demand gives released energy a direction. Without demand, availability can remain only availability. The system may have fuel present, but fuel becomes meaningful only when it is matched to tissue-level work.

The body's demand for energy is continuous and layered. Movement requires energy, but movement is only one expression of demand. Organs require energy. The brain requires energy. Temperature regulation requires energy. Tissue repair requires energy. Immune activity requires energy. Digestion, circulation, cellular maintenance, and ordinary daily function all require ongoing energy flow.

Because demand exists at multiple levels, utilization should not be reduced to workouts or formal activity. The body is always using energy to remain organized and functional. Released fat-derived energy may contribute to that broader demand when conditions support its use.

Movement can increase tissue demand, making circulating fuel more relevant. Ordinary daily output, posture, walking, work tasks, household movement, and structured activity all contribute to the energy environment. But demand is not automatically beneficial simply because it increases. Demand must still be integrated with recovery capacity and system stability.

If movement demand rises beyond what the system can recover from, compensation can increase. Fatigue may rise. Appetite pressure may intensify. Spontaneous movement may fall. Stress signaling may increase. Recovery demand may become more prominent. In that environment, released energy may still be used, but the system may also respond in ways that reduce continuity or increase compensatory pressure.

This is why utilization belongs inside a stability framework rather than an intensity framework. The relevant question is not simply whether demand exists. Demand always exists. The more precise question is whether released energy can be used within a coordinated system without creating compensation that overwhelms continuity.

Fuel use also depends on the system's ability to shift among available fuels. This is where metabolic flexibility becomes important.

Metabolic flexibility refers to the capacity to adjust fuel use according to availability and demand. The body may rely more heavily on glucose in some conditions, glycogen in others, fat-derived energy in others, and mixed fuel use across many ordinary states. Fuel selection is not fixed. It changes with feeding status, activity demand, stress signals, sleep state, hormonal coordination, recovery status, and tissue needs.

When fuel transitions are coordinated, utilization can become more stable. Released fat-derived energy can contribute more effectively when tissues can shift toward using it under appropriate conditions. When fuel transitions are less coordinated, released energy may not become functional output as smoothly. Mobilization may occur, but use may be less consistent.

This does not turn metabolic flexibility into an optimization target in this chapter. It simply clarifies that released energy must fit into the system's current fuel-use pattern. The body does not use every available fuel equally at all times. It selects and prioritizes according to context.

At the tissue level, released fuel must also be processed into usable energy. Mitochondria can be understood here in broad systems terms as energy-processing structures within cells. They are part of the machinery that converts available fuel into functional output. Detailed biochemistry is not necessary for the central point: release from storage is not the same as tissue-level use.

A fuel can be available in circulation without being processed into useful work at the required rate. Utilization depends not only on access and mobilization, but also on whether tissues can receive and process the available fuel within the demands of the current state.

This introduces another layer of the pathway. Stored energy must be accessible. It must be mobilized. It must circulate. Then tissues must be able to use it. Each stage matters because fat loss depends on the sequence continuing across time.

Competing fuel availability can influence that sequence. If glucose, glycogen, or incoming nutrients are readily available, mobilized fat-derived energy may not be prioritized to the same degree. This does not mean mobilization failed. It means the system is choosing among available fuels according to context.

The body often has multiple energy sources available at once. Incoming nutrients may be present after feeding. Glycogen may provide shorter-term reserve energy. Glucose may be prioritized under certain demands. Fat-derived energy may be more relevant in other conditions. The system coordinates among these sources rather than treating mobilized fat as automatically dominant once it appears.

Fat loss becomes more meaningful when mobilized energy is used consistently enough over time to reduce stored reserves. Temporary use may occur without producing a large visible change. Temporary mobilization may occur without becoming sustained utilization. The pattern matters because stored-energy reduction is cumulative.

Recovery and stress shape the environment in which utilization occurs.

Poor recovery can reduce movement output, increase fatigue, alter appetite pressure, disrupt glucose stability, and narrow the system's ability to coordinate energy use. A system with limited recovery capacity may still mobilize and use fuel, but the process may occur with more compensation. The body may respond by lowering output, increasing intake pressure, or shifting priorities toward repair and conservation.

Stress can alter glucose availability, hormonal coordination, fluid balance, substrate preference, and perceived energy demand. It does not simply "block" utilization. That framing is too crude. Stress changes the environment in which released energy is processed. Under higher strain, the system may prioritize immediate availability, glucose support, vigilance, or recovery-related demands in ways that alter the role of mobilized fat-derived energy.

These influences do not make fat loss impossible. They explain why utilization is conditional.

Released energy is used within an environment shaped by demand, fuel availability, tissue capacity, stress load, recovery state, hormonal coordination, and broader system stability. No single factor completes the process alone.

This chapter's mechanism defines the gap between release and use.

The Mobilization–Utilization Gap Mechanism states that fat released from storage does not become meaningful fat loss unless the system uses it over time.

The first side of the mechanism is mobilization. Energy moves out of storage and becomes more available.

The second side is utilization. Tissues use that energy to support function across time.

The gap between these stages explains why short-term release does not automatically equal durable fat loss. Mobilization may occur without enough sustained use to reduce stored reserves meaningfully. Utilization is the stage where released energy becomes part of functional output rather than remaining only a circulating possibility.

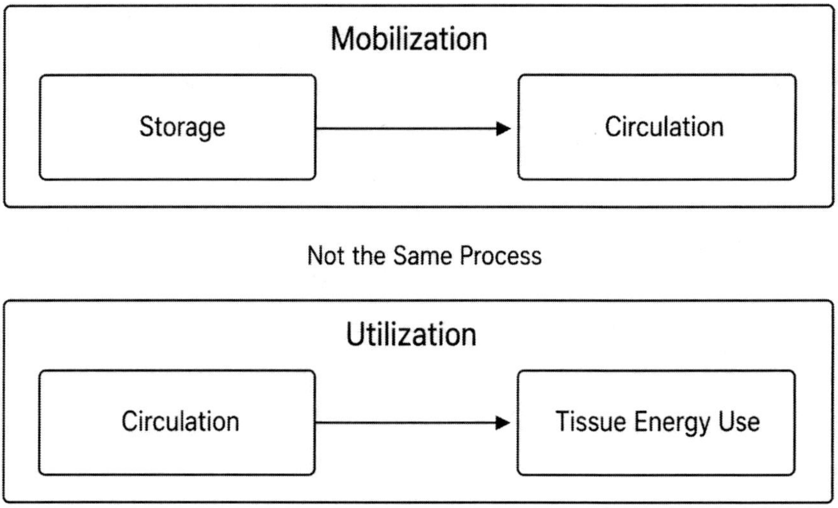

[Figure 6: Mobilization vs Utilization Model]

The figure separates two connected but distinct stages. The first stage, mobilization, moves energy from storage to circulation. The second stage, utilization, moves energy from circulation into tissue energy use. The gap between them is labeled because these are not the same process. Fat loss depends on the sequence continuing across time, not merely on the first stage occurring.

This model prevents the pathway from being compressed into a single event. Access is not mobilization. Mobilization is not utilization. Utilization is not automatically durable fat loss unless it persists long enough to reduce the stored reserve. Each stage contributes to the larger outcome, but none should be mistaken for the entire process.

The distinction matters for interpretation. A temporary increase in released fat-derived energy does not necessarily produce visible or durable reduction. The system may mobilize energy under certain conditions, use some of it, displace some of it, or return some of it toward storage. The outcome depends on the broader pattern across time.

This is why short-term "fat-burning" language is imprecise. It often refers to a momentary shift in substrate use or mobilization, then implies that meaningful stored-energy reduction has occurred. But fat loss stability depends on sustained coordination, not temporary emphasis on one fuel source.

Access, mobilization, and utilization must remain connected long enough to change the reserve.

This first pathway gives the rest of the book its structure. Stored fat must become accessible before it can leave storage. Mobilized energy must be directed toward use rather than only circulation or re-storage. Utilized energy must contribute to functional output over time before stored reserves decline in a meaningful way.

Once this pathway is established, the next question becomes how the body regulates it.

Insulin is one of the major signals involved in coordinating storage, access, and use. It influences whether incoming energy is stored, whether stored energy is released, and how the system interprets current availability. But insulin must be understood as regulation, not as a villain or single controller.

Fat loss is not complete when energy leaves storage. It becomes meaningful when released energy is used within a coordinated system over time.

Insulin and the Regulation of Stored Energy

The previous chapters established the first major pathway of fat loss. Stored energy must become accessible before it can leave reserve status. Once accessible, it can be mobilized into circulation. Once mobilized, it must be used by tissues over time before meaningful reduction of stored reserves occurs.

The next question is how the body regulates movement through that pathway.

Insulin is one of the major signals involved in that regulation.

Few metabolic signals are discussed in more simplified or polarized ways than insulin. In some interpretations, insulin is treated as if it single-handedly determines fat loss and permanently blocks access to stored energy whenever it rises. In other interpretations, insulin is treated as largely irrelevant, with no meaningful role in storage or fuel regulation at all. Both positions flatten a coordinated system into a single-variable argument.

Insulin matters, but it matters as part of a broader regulatory environment.

The body does not use insulin as a moral signal or a punishment signal. It uses insulin as a coordination signal. Insulin helps interpret incoming energy and organize what happens afterward. It participates in nutrient uptake, storage direction, fuel partitioning, circulation, and access to stored reserves. Its role is not to "cause" fat loss or "prevent" fat loss in isolation. Its role is to help coordinate how energy moves through the system under changing conditions.

This distinction becomes easier to understand once fat loss is viewed as a sequence rather than a single event. Chapters 4 through 6 established that stored energy must move through several stages before stored reserves decline meaningfully. Access, mobilization, and utilization all occur within a regulated environment. Insulin is one of the signals shaping that environment.

After food enters the system, insulin helps coordinate nutrient handling. Glucose moves into tissues. Glycogen storage is supported. Incoming energy becomes available for immediate use, short-term reserve, or longer-term storage depending on current demand and availability. This coordination reduces the need to rely heavily on stored reserves when incoming fuel is already present.

Storage is therefore not dysfunction. It is one normal metabolic direction.

The body stores energy because future demand and future intake are not always synchronized. Insulin participates in the handling of incoming energy so that nutrients can be directed appropriately rather than remaining uncontrolled in circulation. Without this coordination, the system would struggle to maintain glucose stability, tissue uptake, and organized energy distribution.

This is why insulin cannot be understood accurately through purely oppositional language. The body requires insulin for nutrient handling, glucose regulation, tissue uptake, and energy continuity. The question for fat loss is not whether insulin is "good" or "bad." The more precise question is how insulin signaling influences the conditions under which stored energy becomes more or less available.

Insulin tone influences whether the system relies more heavily on incoming energy or stored reserves at a given moment.

When insulin tone is higher, the system generally favors uptake, storage, and use of incoming energy while reducing reliance on long-term reserves. The body interprets available incoming fuel as sufficient for at least part of current demand. Under those conditions, release from stored fat tends to become less emphasized because energy is already entering the system from another source.

When insulin tone is lower, stored-energy access may become more permissive. The system may rely more heavily on reserve energy because incoming energy handling becomes less dominant relative to current demand.

But this relationship should not be simplified into a direct formula where lower insulin automatically equals fat loss.

Access is only one stage of the pathway. Stored energy may become more available while mobilization, utilization, recovery state, stress load, competing fuel availability, or system stability still influence the overall outcome. A system can permit greater access without necessarily producing stable or durable reduction in stored reserves.

This is one reason single-variable explanations of fat loss repeatedly become incomplete. The body is not responding only to insulin. It is coordinating multiple signals simultaneously. Demand matters. Recovery matters. Stress matters. Glucose behavior matters. Activity state matters. Appetite regulation matters. Fuel competition matters. Insulin participates in that larger environment rather than replacing it.

The role of insulin becomes clearer when viewed through fuel partitioning.

Fuel partitioning refers to how the body directs available energy toward different destinations. Incoming nutrients may be used immediately, stored temporarily as glycogen, stored longer-term as fat, circulated for current demand, or held in reserve depending on conditions. Insulin helps coordinate these directional priorities.

This connects directly to the earlier chapters.

Stored energy must become accessible before it can leave reserve status. Mobilized energy must move into circulation. Circulating energy must be used by tissues. Insulin influences the conditions surrounding those transitions because it helps shape whether incoming energy handling or stored-energy reliance becomes more dominant under current conditions.

When incoming energy is plentiful and insulin tone remains elevated accordingly, the body generally reduces emphasis on drawing from long-term reserves. When incoming energy handling becomes less dominant, stored-energy access may increase if the broader environment supports it.

Again, this does not make insulin a wall separating the body from stored fat. The system is more dynamic than that. Stored energy can still be mobilized under a range of insulin conditions because regulation is continuous rather than binary. The relevant distinction is directional emphasis. Higher insulin tone generally shifts priority toward uptake and storage-related processes. Lower insulin tone generally permits greater access to stored reserves.

But insulin signaling never acts in isolation.

A person may experience conditions permissive to stored-energy access while still lacking sufficient demand or utilization for meaningful reduction to occur. Released energy may circulate without being used strongly enough over time to lower the reserve substantially. Similarly, a person may experience high stress load, poor recovery, unstable sleep, increased appetite pressure, or reduced movement output that alters the broader fat-loss environment independently of insulin alone.

This is why insulin-centered explanations often become distorted when they attempt to explain the entire metabolic system through one signal.

Insulin matters because it helps coordinate energy handling. It does not replace every other layer of regulation.

The body's energy environment remains multi-variable even when insulin signaling is central to the discussion. Access, mobilization, utilization, recovery capacity, appetite regulation, glucose stability, stress exposure, and output demand continue interacting simultaneously.

This chapter's mechanism emerges from that broader framing.

The Insulin Constraint Mechanism states that insulin helps regulate whether energy is being stored, accessed, circulated, or used.

The mechanism contains two connected sides.

The first is storage coordination. Insulin helps direct incoming energy toward uptake and storage. Nutrients entering circulation after feeding are coordinated into tissues and reserve systems according to current conditions and demand. This supports glucose regulation, glycogen replenishment, tissue uptake, and broader energy stability.

The second is access constraint. Insulin tone helps influence whether stored energy remains more protected or becomes more available. Higher insulin tone generally reduces emphasis on reserve release. Lower insulin tone may permit greater stored-energy access depending on the surrounding environment.

Constraint here does not mean obstruction or opposition. It means regulatory boundary.

Insulin helps shape the conditions under which stored energy becomes more or less available. The signal influences directionality within the energy system rather than functioning as an all-or-nothing barrier.

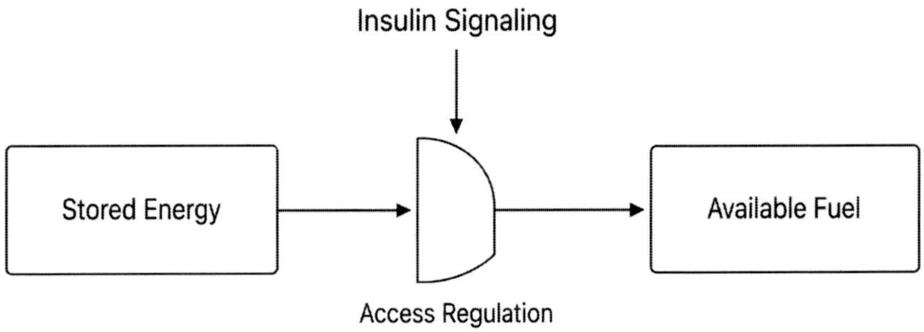

[Figure 7: Insulin and Stored Energy Access]

The figure presents stored energy on one side and available fuel on the other, with access regulation positioned between them. Insulin signaling appears above the regulatory checkpoint because insulin influences the conditions surrounding access rather than acting as a simple on-off switch. The gate is intentionally shown as partially regulated rather than completely open or closed. Stored energy can become more or less available depending on insulin tone and the broader state of the system.

The figure also reinforces that insulin is not operating independently from context. Incoming energy availability, activity demand, stress state, recovery quality, competing fuels, and overall metabolic coordination continue influencing how the access environment behaves. Insulin participates in regulating the pathway rather than dictating it alone.

This distinction matters because fat loss stability depends on coordinated regulation rather than isolated activation of one variable.

A system with lower insulin tone may still experience unstable appetite regulation, poor recovery, insufficient utilization, or high compensatory pressure that limits durable reduction of stored reserves. Conversely, a system may maintain relatively stable fat loss despite periods of higher insulin signaling if broader coordination among access, demand, utilization, and recovery remains intact.

The pathway remains integrated.

Instability tends to emerge when incoming energy handling, stored-energy access, glucose behavior, appetite pressure, movement output, stress signaling, and recovery capacity become poorly coordinated relative to one another. Under those conditions, the system may produce compensation, volatility, fluctuating energy availability, or inconsistent movement through the access–mobilization–utilization sequence.

Insulin participates in that coordination because it helps regulate fuel direction and nutrient handling across changing states. But the body's overall energy behavior still depends on multiple overlapping signals interacting continuously.

This is also why insulin discussions often drift into false binary thinking. One side attempts to explain all fat loss through insulin alone. The other attempts to remove insulin from the conversation almost entirely. Both approaches reduce a regulatory system into ideological simplification.

The more accurate systems view is narrower and more precise.

Insulin is one of the major signals influencing whether energy is stored, accessed, circulated, or used. It helps coordinate transitions between incoming energy and stored energy. It influences how strongly the system relies on immediate fuel versus reserve fuel under current conditions. But the outcome of fat loss still depends on whether stored energy ultimately becomes accessible, mobilized, utilized, and sustained within a stable enough environment for reserves to decline across time.

This chapter therefore positions insulin where it belongs: important, influential, but not solitary.

The next chapter widens the hormonal frame further. Insulin is not the entire signaling environment regulating fat loss. Appetite-related signals, stress-related signals, counter-regulatory signals, recovery-related signals, and broader hormonal coordination all influence how the body interprets energy availability and future demand.

Fat loss is not governed by one isolated signal. It emerges from coordinated regulation across systems. Insulin should therefore be understood not as the enemy of fat loss, but as part of the regulatory environment determining how energy moves between storage, availability, circulation, and use.

Hormonal Coordination Beyond Insulin

Chapter 7 established insulin as one of the major signals involved in stored-energy regulation. Insulin helps coordinate whether energy is being stored, accessed, circulated, or used. It influences the conditions surrounding reserve protection and fuel availability, but insulin does not represent the entire hormonal environment.

The body does not regulate stored energy through one signal alone.

Fat loss is often oversimplified by assigning too much explanatory power to a single hormone at a time. One framework elevates insulin. Another centers cortisol. Another emphasizes thyroid signaling. Another focuses almost entirely on hunger hormones or reproductive hormones. Each model identifies something real, but then expands that single signal into a complete explanation.

The systems view is narrower and more precise.

These signals matter because they participate in regulation. They influence how the body interprets energy availability, recovery demand, stress exposure, appetite pressure, reserve security, and current output requirements. But they do not operate independently from one another. Fat loss emerges from coordinated signaling across systems rather than from one dominant switch controlling the entire process.

Hormones should therefore be understood here as regulatory signals shaping the energy environment.

The point is not that every hormone directly causes fat gain or fat loss in a simple linear way. The point is that multiple signaling systems influence the conditions under which stored energy is protected, released, circulated, or used. These signals help determine whether the body emphasizes immediate availability, reserve protection, energy turnover, recovery, vigilance, or longer-horizon continuity under current conditions.

Stress-related signaling is one part of that environment.

Stress signals influence glucose availability, substrate preference, vigilance, fluid balance, appetite pressure, and recovery demand. Under changing stress conditions, the body may shift toward shorter-horizon energy priorities. Immediate availability may become more important than smooth reserve reduction. Appetite signals may become more intense. Sleep quality may become less stable. Recovery demand may increase. Fuel use patterns may shift toward maintaining readiness rather than preserving long-term consistency.

This does not mean stress hormones simply "block fat loss." That explanation compresses a complex adaptive response into a single outcome claim. Stress-related signaling changes the conditions under which energy is regulated. It alters how the system interprets uncertainty, workload, recovery needs, and future availability. Under higher strain, the body may regulate stored energy differently because the broader operating environment has changed.

Thyroid-related signaling shapes another part of the environment.

Thyroid signaling helps influence metabolic rate, temperature regulation, tissue activity, and general energy throughput. It contributes to how much energy the system is moving and how actively tissues are operating. This does not mean thyroid signaling directly "burns fat." It means the overall pace and turnover of energy processing are influenced by thyroid-related coordination.

Fat loss therefore occurs within a broader throughput environment. A system moving energy rapidly, maintaining tissue activity efficiently, and supporting stable turnover behaves differently from a system operating with lower throughput, reduced activity, or constrained energy movement. The relevant distinction is not whether thyroid signaling alone determines fat loss. The distinction is that energy release and energy use occur within a system whose overall pace and operating intensity are partly shaped by thyroid-related regulation.

Hunger and satiety signaling add another layer of coordination.

Signals related to hunger, fullness, food reward, energy sufficiency, and intake urgency influence the pressure surrounding food-seeking behavior and energy acquisition. These signals are often treated culturally as measures of discipline or self-control, but within a systems framework they are regulatory communication.

Appetite signals help the body interpret current and future energy conditions. Hunger intensity may rise when energy availability appears uncertain, when stress load increases, when sleep becomes unstable, or when reserve reduction persists long enough to increase perceived energy urgency. Satiety signaling may shift according to energy density, nutrient availability, recovery status, glucose behavior, and broader hormonal coordination.

These signals influence the fat-loss environment because they affect continuity. Fat loss depends on conditions supporting reserve reduction across time. Appetite regulation helps determine whether those conditions remain stable or become increasingly difficult to sustain.

Reproductive signaling influences energy allocation in another way.

Reproductive hormones participate in fertility-related priorities, tissue state, recovery interpretation, energy sufficiency assessment, and cycle-dependent variability. The body does not separate reproductive state from energy regulation. Reserve availability, recovery capacity, and perceived energy security all interact with reproductive signaling.

This chapter is not attempting to build a sex-specific hormone framework or explain reproductive endocrinology in detail. The broader systems point is simpler. Reproductive state influences how the body interprets energy conditions. Under some circumstances, the system may place greater emphasis on reserve security, recovery support, or energy continuity because reproductive signaling forms part of the larger regulatory environment.

Sleep-related signaling widens the frame further because sleep affects several systems simultaneously.

Sleep quality and circadian alignment influence glucose regulation, appetite signaling, stress response, nervous system state, recovery quality, and energy stability. Sleep disruption does not alter only one variable. It changes coordination across multiple regulatory systems at once.

When sleep quality deteriorates, appetite pressure may increase. Stress signaling may become more prominent. Recovery quality may decline. Glucose behavior may become less stable. Fatigue may alter movement output and energy demand. The result is not a single isolated effect on fat loss. The result is a broader change in the environment through which stored energy is regulated.

Sleep-related signaling matters because coordinated systems tend to regulate energy more coherently than disrupted systems. Recovery, appetite, stress response, and energy use all become harder to align when sleep-related regulation becomes unstable.

Nervous system state adds another level of interpretation.

The nervous system influences vigilance, arousal, recovery tone, rest state, energy direction, and physiological readiness. A system operating under higher sympathetic pressure may allocate energy differently from one operating with stronger parasympathetic recovery support. Under higher vigilance, the body may emphasize readiness, immediate availability, and rapid response. Under stronger recovery support, restoration, repair, digestion, and longer-horizon coordination may become more prominent.

Neither state is inherently good or bad. Both are necessary parts of regulation. The issue for fat loss stability is whether the system can coordinate between demand and recovery without remaining trapped in prolonged instability.

Nervous system state interacts with stress response, appetite behavior, sleep quality, recovery capacity, and fuel use patterns. It influences the environment in which stored-energy access and utilization occur rather than functioning as an isolated mechanism by itself.

These signaling systems overlap continuously.

Stress affects sleep. Sleep affects appetite. Appetite affects intake behavior and perceived energy urgency. Reproductive signaling influences recovery and energy interpretation. Thyroid-related signaling affects throughput and turnover. Nervous system state interacts with vigilance, restoration, and stress response. Insulin interacts with incoming energy handling and stored-energy access.

The body therefore regulates stored energy through coordinated interaction rather than isolated control.

This is the chapter's central mechanism.

The Hormonal Coordination Mechanism states that fat loss depends on coordinated signaling across multiple regulatory systems, not a single switch.

The first side of the mechanism is multiple regulatory inputs. Several hormonal and signaling systems influence the fat-loss environment simultaneously. Stress-related signals, insulin signaling, thyroid-related coordination, appetite-related signals, reproductive signals, sleep-related regulation, and nervous system state all contribute to how the body interprets current and future energy conditions.

The second side is coordinated outcome. Stored-energy release and reduction depend on how these signals interact. Fat loss does not emerge because one hormone becomes dominant. It emerges when the overall signaling environment supports stable access, release, utilization, appetite regulation, recovery, and continuity strongly enough for stored reserves to decline across time.

The central question is therefore not which hormone matters most. The more useful question is whether the signaling environment is coordinated well enough to support stable energy regulation without excessive compensation, instability, or reserve protection pressure.

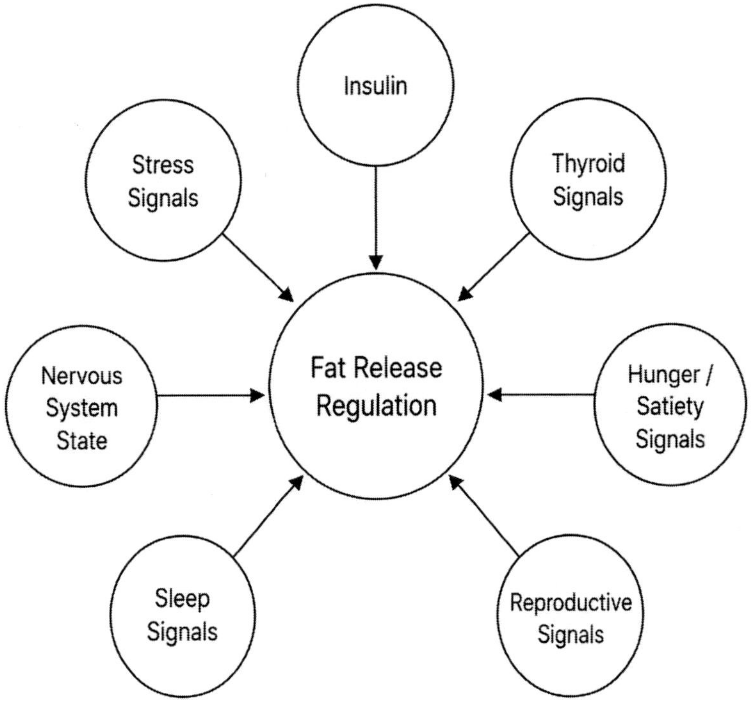

[Figure 8: Hormonal Signals Governing Fat Release]

The figure places fat release regulation at the center and surrounds it with multiple signaling inputs. Insulin appears alongside stress signals, thyroid-related signals, hunger and satiety signals, sleep-related signals, reproductive signals, and nervous system state. Thin arrows connect each regulatory input to the central process because fat release is influenced by overlapping communication rather than isolated command.

The diagram prevents the reader from collapsing the chapter into a single-hormone explanation. No signal appears as the master controller. Instead, the figure shows that stored-energy regulation occurs within a broader network of interacting systems. The body interprets energy conditions through combined signaling patterns rather than through one isolated variable.

This matters for fat loss stability because stable reserve reduction depends on coordination rather than contradiction.

When appetite pressure, stress signaling, recovery quality, glucose behavior, energy turnover, and nervous system state remain relatively aligned, the conditions supporting stored-energy release and use become easier to sustain across time. When these systems begin operating at cross-purposes, instability tends to increase. In that environment, access, mobilization, and utilization may still occur, but they are less likely to remain coordinated long enough to support stable reserve reduction.

A person may experience elevated appetite pressure while recovery declines. Stress signaling may increase while sleep quality worsens. Energy turnover may slow while fatigue reduces movement output. Glucose behavior may become more volatile while nervous system arousal remains elevated. Under those conditions, stored-energy release may become less stable not because one hormone "failed," but because the signaling environment has become poorly coordinated.

This distinction also prevents hormone panic frameworks from taking over the discussion.

The body is not governed by a single defective switch waiting to be corrected. Hormonal regulation is dynamic, adaptive, and interactive. Fat loss occurs within that broader adaptive environment rather than outside it.

The next chapter moves from signaling toward balance. Once multiple systems influencing release are understood, the next question becomes how storage and release interact over time. Fat loss does not occur because storage mechanisms disappear completely. Storage remains part of normal metabolic regulation. Fat loss occurs when release and use exceed storage across time within a coordinated system.

Fat loss should therefore not be explained through one hormone in isolation. It is better understood as the outcome of coordinated regulation across multiple interacting systems.

Storage and Release Are Always in Balance

Chapter 8 widened the regulatory frame beyond insulin by showing that fat release is influenced by multiple signaling systems. Stress-related signals, thyroid-related signaling, appetite signals, reproductive signals, sleep-related regulation, and nervous system state all shape the conditions under which stored energy becomes more protected, more accessible, or more difficult to reduce consistently.

But release is only one side of the larger process.

The body is always managing both storage and release. Energy regulation does not operate as a simple switch flipped from storage to fat loss. The body can store some energy while releasing other energy across different tissues, timeframes, and conditions. Incoming nutrients can be directed toward immediate use, short-term storage, or longer-term reserve while stored energy is also being mobilized and used elsewhere.

This makes binary thinking misleading. Fat loss does not require storage to disappear completely. Storage is not the opposite of fat loss in a moral or mechanical sense. It is one normal direction of energy handling. Release is also normal, but release alone does not prove that stored reserves are declining across time.

Both processes remain active. The question is which direction dominates over the longer interval.

Storage occurs because incoming energy must be handled. After feeding, the body may direct available energy toward current tissue needs, glycogen storage, circulating availability, or longer-term reserve. This is not failure. It is coordination. Energy entering the system has to be distributed somewhere, and storage is part of how the body preserves continuity across future demand.

Release occurs when stored energy becomes accessible, mobilized, circulated, and used under conditions that support reserve use. This process allows the body to draw from prior storage when current demand, incoming energy, and regulatory signals make stored reserves relevant.

Neither process is inherently good or bad. Storage and release are regulatory directions.

Fat loss reflects the net direction of their relationship over time. Stored reserves decline when release and use exceed storage and re-storage across a meaningful interval. The body may still store energy at certain moments during a period when longer-term stored reserves are decreasing. The key is not whether storage ever occurs. The key is whether more stored energy leaves reserve and is used than enters or returns to reserve across time.

This is important because fat loss does not place the body into a permanent release-only condition. The system still has to handle incoming nutrients, maintain glucose availability, refill short-term reserves, and preserve energy for future demand. Even during a longer period of stored-reserve reduction, the body may temporarily direct energy into storage when conditions call for it. That temporary storage does not automatically contradict the larger trend. It simply reflects the fact that energy handling continues while fat mass changes slowly across time.

Timescale is therefore central.

Short-term storage can occur within a longer-term fat-loss trend. A meal may produce incoming energy that is temporarily stored while the broader direction of stored reserves continues downward across days or weeks. A short-term release event can also occur without long-term fat loss if later storage offsets it. A period of mobilization does not guarantee durable reduction if the released energy is not used consistently enough or if later conditions return energy to reserve.

This prevents over-interpretation of isolated moments.

The body is always moving through smaller cycles inside larger trends. A single meal, a single fast, a single workout, or a single day of lower intake may shift the balance temporarily, but none of those moments reveals the full direction of stored reserves by itself. The longer pattern matters because fat mass changes through accumulated direction, not isolated metabolic snapshots. Short-term events can influence the balance, but they do not replace the balance.

A single meal does not define the entire storage–release balance. A single workout does not prove stored reserves are declining. A fasting interval does not guarantee durable fat loss. A single day of scale movement does not reveal the net direction of fat mass. These events matter only as part of the longer relationship between storage pressure and release-and-use pressure.

This distinction is necessary because fat-loss culture often treats the body as if it has two modes: storing or losing. That framing collapses a continuous regulatory process into a binary state. It also makes ordinary storage feel like interruption and ordinary release feel like completion.

Neither interpretation is precise.

The body can be handling incoming energy while still trending toward stored-reserve reduction over time. It can also release stored energy temporarily while the larger pattern remains neutral or storage-dominant. Fat loss stability depends on the long-term relationship between these directions, not on the elimination of one side.

The access–mobilization–utilization pathway from Chapters 4 through 6 fits directly into this balance. Release matters only when stored energy becomes accessible, leaves storage, enters circulation, and is used by tissues. Access opens the reserve. Mobilization moves energy out of storage.

Utilization turns released energy into functional output. Together, these stages create release-and-use pressure.

Storage pressure operates in the opposite direction. Incoming energy may enter reserve. Circulating energy may return toward storage. Mobilized energy that is not used may be re-stored. Storage pressure is therefore not limited to obvious accumulation. It includes any pathway by which energy enters or returns to reserve.

This includes mobilized energy that does not remain on a path toward use. When released energy is not needed, when competing fuels are more available, or when demand falls relative to availability, some of that energy may return toward storage. This does not mean the original mobilization was meaningless. It means release and final reduction are separated by conditions that determine where energy goes next. The same stored reserve can be opened, partially drawn upon, and partially refilled as the system continues regulating availability.

The long-term direction of fat mass depends on the relationship between these pathways.

Insulin and hormonal coordination influence that relationship. Insulin helps coordinate incoming energy handling, nutrient uptake, storage, and stored-energy access. Higher insulin tone generally favors incoming energy handling and reduced reliance on long-term reserves, while lower insulin tone may permit greater access depending on the broader system state.

But insulin does not determine the entire balance by itself. Broader hormonal signaling shapes appetite pressure, stress response, sleep quality, recovery demand, energy turnover, reproductive priorities, nervous system state, and fuel use. These signals influence whether storage pressure or release-and-use pressure becomes more dominant across time.

Demand also matters. When tissues require energy, release-and-use pressure may become more relevant. But demand must be integrated with recovery. Excessive demand relative to recovery capacity can increase compensation, appetite pressure, fatigue, or stress load, altering the same balance it was expected to shift.

Incoming energy matters because storage pressure cannot be understood without considering what enters the system. But incoming energy is still interpreted through regulation. The body handles nutrients according to current demand, fuel availability, hormonal signaling, recovery state, and reserve status.

Recovery matters because coordinated release and use require system stability. Poor recovery can reduce output, increase appetite pressure, disrupt glucose behavior, and shift the storage–release environment toward compensation or conservation.

The Storage–Release Balance Mechanism defines the chapter's central claim: fat loss reflects a long-term shift in the balance between stored energy entering and leaving reserve.

The mechanism has two sides.

The first side is storage pressure. Energy enters or returns to reserve. This can occur through incoming energy being stored, mobilized energy being re-stored, or conditions favoring reserve protection and accumulation.

The second side is release-and-use pressure. Stored energy becomes accessible, mobilized, and utilized. This is the pathway through which reserve energy leaves storage and contributes to functional output.

Fat loss does not require storage pressure to disappear completely. It requires release-and-use pressure to exceed storage pressure over time.

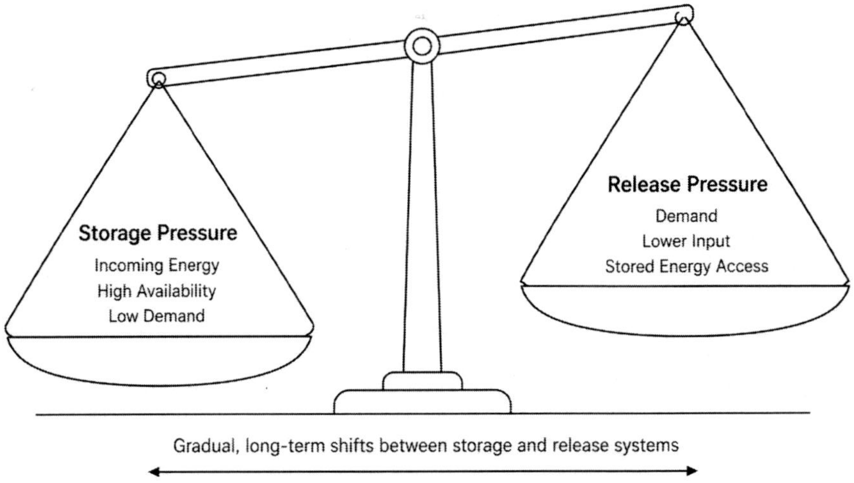

[Figure 9: Storage and Release Balance]

The figure shows storage and release as competing but continuously active pressures. One side represents storage pressure through incoming energy, high availability, and low demand. The other side represents release pressure through demand, lower input, and stored-energy access. The scale is tilted to show directional balance rather than complete dominance. Fat loss occurs when the balance shifts toward release and use across time.

The figure should not be interpreted as one side vanishing. Storage remains part of metabolism. Release remains part of metabolism. The direction of stored reserves depends on how these pressures relate across time.

This model prevents "storage off / fat loss on" thinking.

The body does not need to eliminate storage in order to reduce stored reserves. It needs the long-term balance to favor release and use. A single storage-supportive moment does not erase a longer trend, and a single release-supportive moment does not prove durable fat loss.

This distinction improves interpretation because it removes unnecessary drama from ordinary metabolic events. Feeding, storage, release, mobilization, and use are all normal processes. Fat loss is not the heroic victory of one process over another. It is the net result of their regulated relationship across time.

Chapter 10 will build from this balance model by examining the deficit signal. Once storage and release are understood as active pressures, a deficit can be explained more accurately. A deficit is not a command that forces fat to disappear. It is a condition that changes incoming energy, output demand, and regulatory interpretation. It can shift the storage–release environment, but the body still responds through access, mobilization, utilization, appetite, recovery, stress signaling, and compensation.

Fat loss is not a switch.

It is a long-term shift in the direction of an active balance.

The Deficit Signal

Chapter 9 established that fat loss reflects the long-term relationship between storage pressure and release-and-use pressure. Stored reserves decline when more energy leaves reserve and is used than enters or returns to storage across time. The body is continuously managing both directions. Storage does not disappear during fat loss, and release alone does not guarantee long-term reserve reduction.

The deficit matters because it can shift this balance.

Reduced incoming energy may increase reliance on stored reserves by changing the relationship between current availability and current demand. When less incoming energy is present relative to what the system is using, stored energy can become more relevant as a reserve source. This is why the concept of deficit remains central to fat loss. Stored reserves cannot decline meaningfully if incoming energy and returning storage consistently exceed release and use.

But the deficit does not act as a direct command.

Fat loss discussions often treat reduced intake as if the body receives a mathematical instruction: less energy enters, therefore stored energy must decline in exact proportion. This framing captures part of the energy relationship, but it removes biological interpretation from the process. The body does not experience a deficit as arithmetic alone. It experiences reduced incoming energy as a change in availability that must be interpreted, regulated, and managed across multiple systems.

Arithmetic describes the relationship between incoming energy, outgoing energy, and stored reserves. Signal describes the body's response to changed availability.

Both matter, but they are not the same.

This distinction is what allows the deficit to be taken seriously without being treated as complete explanation. The deficit describes pressure on the storage–release balance, but pressure is not the same as outcome. The body still determines how that pressure is expressed through access, appetite, output, recovery, stress response, and adaptation. Reduced incoming energy may create the conditions for stored reserves to become more relevant, but the stability of that process depends on how the system responds once that pressure appears.

The arithmetic side explains why stored reserves become relevant when incoming energy decreases relative to demand. The signaling side explains why the same apparent deficit can produce different physiological and behavioral responses under different conditions. A deficit changes the environment inside which storage, release, appetite, recovery, output, and adaptation are regulated.

This distinction matters because two situations with similar numerical intake reduction can produce very different experiences and outcomes depending on the broader system state.

A deficit occurring under stable sleep, manageable stress, sufficient recovery, coherent meal structure, tolerable demand, and relatively stable glucose behavior may be interpreted differently from a deficit occurring during fragmented sleep, elevated stress load, unstable glucose patterns, excessive recovery burden, repeated prior restriction, or high appetite pressure.

The numerical relationship may appear similar while the biological response differs substantially.

This does not mean energy relationships disappear. It means the body interprets those relationships through regulation rather than through spreadsheet logic alone.

The body responds to reduced incoming energy through multiple pathways simultaneously. Stored-energy access may increase. Appetite pressure may rise. Output may change. Recovery demands may become more difficult to support. Stress-related signaling may shift. Adaptation may begin to emerge if reduced availability persists long enough.

These responses are not signs that the arithmetic became irrelevant. They are signs that the body is regulating around altered conditions.

Sleep is one of the major variables shaping how reduced incoming energy is experienced. Sleep influences appetite regulation, glucose behavior, stress response, recovery quality, cognitive function, and energy output. When sleep becomes unstable, reduced intake may feel more difficult even if the external deficit appears unchanged. Appetite urgency may increase. Fatigue may rise. Recovery quality may decline. Output may become less stable.

This does not mean poor sleep mechanically prevents fat loss. It means sleep changes the regulatory environment through which the deficit is interpreted.

Stress also alters the environment surrounding reduced intake. Stress-related signaling influences glucose availability, vigilance, fluid regulation, substrate preference, appetite pressure, and perceived energy urgency. Under higher stress load, the body may prioritize immediate availability and short-term function differently from periods of relative stability.

Again, this should not be reduced to simplistic claims that stress "blocks fat loss." The more precise interpretation is that stress changes how the body responds to reduced incoming energy. The same deficit may feel more tolerable and sustainable under lower stress conditions than under conditions of elevated strain and recovery burden.

Protein availability influences the quality of energy restriction rather than simply the quantity of intake reduction. Protein contributes to tissue support, structural maintenance, satiety signaling, and recovery demands. In the context of reduced incoming energy, protein availability may influence how strongly appetite pressure rises, how well tissues are supported, and how tolerable the deficit feels within the broader system.

This is not a macro prescription. It is part of the biological interpretation layer surrounding reduced intake.

Meal structure also influences how the deficit is experienced. The organization of intake across time can affect appetite rhythm, glucose stability, perceived energy availability, and behavioral continuity. A reduction in intake occurring within relatively coherent feeding patterns may produce different appetite dynamics from a reduction occurring within highly unstable or erratic intake patterns.

The issue is not whether one structure is universally correct. The issue is that the body does not experience reduced intake as a pure number detached from timing, rhythm, predictability, or signal continuity.

Prior dieting exposure can further alter the interpretation environment. Repeated periods of restriction may influence appetite pressure, behavioral expectations, adaptive efficiency, perceived deprivation, and regulatory sensitivity. This should not be framed as irreversible "damage." The body is not broken because it has previously experienced energy restriction. But repeated exposure to aggressive or unstable deficits may influence how future deficits are tolerated and interpreted.

The system carries history forward.

Activity demand shapes how reduced incoming energy interacts with release-and-use pressure. Demand increases the relevance of stored energy because tissues require fuel for movement, repair, thermoregulation, cognition, immune activity, and daily function. But demand cannot be separated from recovery. If activity demand rises beyond recovery capacity while incoming energy remains reduced, compensation pressures may increase through fatigue, appetite, reduced output, or stress signaling.

More demand is not automatically more stable.

Recovery capacity therefore becomes central. Recovery determines how well the system maintains coordination under reduced incoming energy. A deficit tolerated within stable recovery conditions may become far more disruptive when recovery quality declines. Sleep disruption, accumulated stress, excessive demand, unstable intake patterns, or prolonged strain can all reduce the system's ability to maintain continuity while incoming energy remains lower.

Glucose stability also shapes deficit interpretation. Rapid fluctuations in glucose availability can increase hunger, urgency, fatigue, or perceived instability, making the same reduction in intake feel substantially different from a deficit occurring within more stable glucose conditions. The deficit may exist numerically in both situations, but the subjective and physiological environment differs.

Appetite pressure is one of the primary ways the system communicates reduced availability. Hunger, food focus, urgency, cravings, and intake pressure are not simply failures of discipline. They are regulatory outputs influenced by incoming energy, recovery status, glucose behavior, stress load, prior restriction, sleep quality, and energy demand.

A deficit therefore becomes behaviorally relevant through appetite signaling as much as through stored-energy access itself.

The Deficit Signal Mechanism defines the central idea of this chapter: a deficit becomes biologically meaningful when the system interprets reduced incoming energy and responds to it.

The mechanism has two sides.

The first side is reduced incoming energy. This is the external condition that changes the storage–release environment. Less incoming energy relative to demand increases the relevance of stored reserves.

The second side is system interpretation. The body responds through appetite signaling, output regulation, stress response, stored-energy access, mobilization, utilization, recovery adjustments, and adaptation processes. These responses determine whether the deficit produces stable reserve reduction or increasing compensation and instability.

Fat loss depends not only on whether incoming energy is reduced, but on whether the resulting storage–release shift can occur while preserving enough system stability for continuity.

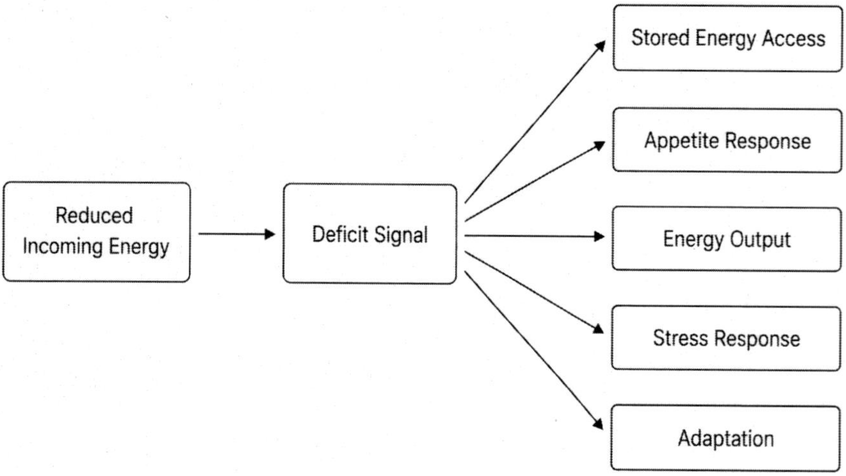

[Figure 10: Calorie Deficit as System Signal]

The figure presents reduced incoming energy as the beginning of a signaling process rather than as a single command. Reduced intake feeds into a central deficit signal, which then branches into multiple system responses: stored-energy access, appetite response, energy output, stress signaling, and adaptation.

This structure matters because it prevents the deficit from being interpreted as a purely mechanical instruction. Reduced incoming energy may increase reliance on stored reserves, but it may also increase appetite pressure, alter recovery demands, influence stress response, and shift output behavior. The body is not merely subtracting energy mathematically. It is reorganizing around altered availability.

This helps explain why deficits vary in stability.

A deficit can support fat loss when the shift toward release and use occurs without creating compensatory pressures strong enough to overwhelm continuity. Stored-energy access may increase while appetite remains manageable, output remains functional, recovery remains adequate, and stress load remains tolerable.

A deficit becomes less stable when the body responds with escalating appetite pressure, declining output, worsening recovery, excessive fatigue, increased stress signaling, or mounting compensation. In those conditions, the same reduction in incoming energy may become progressively harder to sustain because the system is reorganizing around perceived constraint.

This is why fat loss cannot be explained through arithmetic alone even while arithmetic still matters. The energy relationship remains real, but the body interprets that relationship biologically.

The machine analogy fails because machines do not experience hunger, fatigue, adaptation, stress response, or recovery burden. Machines do not alter output in response to reduced availability. Biological systems do.

Chapter 11 will build directly from this point. If reduced incoming energy persists, the system adapts. Adaptation should not be interpreted as panic, damage, or failure. It is the body's attempt to preserve continuity under sustained energy constraint.

The deficit matters because it changes the storage–release environment. But it matters as a signal interpreted by a living system rather than as an instruction executed by a machine.

Adaptation Without Panic

Chapter 10 explained the deficit as a signal rather than a command. Reduced incoming energy changes the storage–release environment, but the body does not respond like a machine executing arithmetic. It interprets reduced availability through appetite, output, stress signaling, recovery demand, stored-energy access, mobilization, utilization, and longer-term regulation.

When that signal persists, the system adapts.

Adaptation is often misunderstood because fat-loss culture tends to use panic language when progress slows. The metabolism is described as broken, damaged, ruined, or resistant. These terms turn ordinary system adjustment into a frightening conclusion. They imply that the body has failed rather than changed.

Panic language also encourages the wrong interpretation of feedback. When a slower rate of change is described as damage, the slowdown becomes evidence of catastrophe rather than evidence of adaptation. The system is treated as if it has lost function, when in many cases it has changed the relationship between intake, output, body mass, recovery demand, and efficiency. This distinction matters because fear-based interpretation tends to produce escalation. More restriction, more activity, or more pressure may be added before the actual mechanism is understood.

A more precise explanation is that the system is no longer operating under the same conditions that existed at the beginning of the deficit.

The body may now have less mass to support. Incoming energy may have been lower for an extended period. Appetite signals may have shifted. Recovery demand may be higher relative to available energy. Movement output may have changed. The original relationship between intake, expenditure, stored energy, and system stability may no longer be the same.

This is adaptation.

Adaptation does not mean nothing can change. It means the conditions producing change have changed. The system adjusts to repeated energy constraint because maintaining function under altered availability requires coordination. A living system does not ignore sustained reduction in incoming energy. It responds by changing output, efficiency, appetite pressure, and allocation.

Body size itself affects energy requirement. A smaller body usually requires less energy to maintain than a larger body because there is less tissue to move, heat, repair, and support. Some reduction in energy expenditure can occur simply because the system being maintained is smaller. This is not malfunction. It is a change in system demand.

That basic change can narrow the original deficit gap. If incoming energy stays the same while body mass decreases, total energy required for maintenance and movement may decline. The gap that was wider at the beginning becomes smaller later because the body itself has changed.

This is one of the simplest forms of adaptation and one of the easiest to misread. A smaller system often requires less energy because there is less tissue to sustain and less mass to move. The reduction in expenditure is not evidence that the system has malfunctioned. It is partly a consequence of the outcome itself. As stored reserves and total body mass change, the energy cost of maintaining and moving the body can change with them. The original deficit was created under one body state. Later, the same pattern is occurring inside a different body state.

Adaptation can also occur through efficiency changes. The system may reduce unnecessary output, conserve movement, lower spontaneous activity, alter fatigue signals, or shift energy allocation toward functions that preserve continuity. None of these responses require conscious intention. They are forms of regulation under repeated constraint.

Spontaneous movement is one place this can appear. The body may produce slightly less non-deliberate movement, less restlessness, less background activity, or lower output across ordinary tasks. Fatigue signals may increase, reducing the tendency toward unnecessary expenditure. These changes may be subtle, but across time they can alter the energy gap that originally supported fat loss.

Subtle changes matter because adaptation does not need to appear dramatic to change the overall balance. Slight reductions in spontaneous movement, task intensity, posture, restlessness, training output, or general daily drive can accumulate across the day. None of these changes may feel like a deliberate choice. They may simply appear as lower motivation, more fatigue, less urgency, or a quieter physical baseline. From the outside, the person may believe the same plan is still being followed. Internally, the system may be spending less energy to preserve continuity under reduced availability.

The same apparent behavior may therefore stop producing the same result. A pattern that created fat loss earlier may later produce slower change because body mass, output, appetite, recovery, and energy allocation have shifted. The external behavior may look similar while the internal system has reorganized around it.

This does not mean the original deficit was imaginary. It means the system adjusted around the deficit.

At the beginning of reduced incoming energy, the gap between intake and expenditure may be relatively wide. Stored reserves may become more relevant, and release-and-use pressure may exceed storage pressure. Over time, body mass decreases, output may decline, efficiency may increase, and appetite pressure may rise. The gap narrows because the system is responding to the conditions it has been experiencing.

This narrowing is often interpreted incorrectly. A slowdown can be framed as failure, resistance, or damage. But a slower rate of change can simply reflect a smaller gap between incoming energy and outgoing energy than existed before. The system has become more efficient or less energetically expensive under the new conditions.

The more precise interpretation is that the original conditions are no longer identical. The early phase of fat loss may include a wider storage–release gap, greater visible movement, and more available margin before compensation rises. Later, the body may be smaller, output may be lower, appetite pressure may be higher, and recovery may be more constrained. The same external pattern can therefore operate with a narrower margin. The slowdown is not proof that the system has stopped responding. It may show that the system has responded enough to change the conditions under which further loss occurs.

Efficiency is not inherently good or bad. It is a description of system behavior.

Under repeated constraint, efficiency can preserve function. The body may require less energy to perform certain tasks or may reduce output that is not immediately necessary. This protects continuity, but it can also make continued fat loss less linear. The same system that allows the body to remain functional under lower availability can narrow the conditions that originally produced faster reserve reduction.

Appetite pressure may also increase as part of adaptation. The system interprets sustained reduced availability and communicates through hunger, food focus, urgency, cravings, or reduced satiety. This is not a moral problem. It is a regulatory response to perceived energy constraint. Chapter 12 will examine compensation more fully, but appetite belongs here as an early sign that the system is adjusting to a repeated signal.

This is important because adaptation is not only metabolic in the narrow sense. It can also change the pressure surrounding behavior. Hunger, food focus, reduced satiety, and increased attention to food can make the same deficit harder to sustain even if the external structure has not changed. The system is not only adjusting expenditure. It is also communicating about availability. That communication becomes one of the bridges between internal adaptation and outward compensation.

Recovery also changes under constraint. When incoming energy remains lower, recovery may become more expensive relative to availability. The body must still allocate energy toward tissue repair, cognition, immune activity, movement, temperature regulation, and daily function. If available energy becomes more limited, the system may prioritize more carefully.

This can make the same deficit feel different over time. Early reduced intake may be tolerated within a wider stability margin. Later, after accumulated stress, lower reserves, smaller body mass, and repeated recovery demands, the same apparent pattern may create more fatigue, more appetite pressure, or slower output.

Stress load interacts with this process. Repeated constraint can become more stressful when recovery capacity is limited. This does not mean every deficit is harmful, nor does it mean adaptation is pathological. It means tolerance for constraint depends on the surrounding system state. Sleep, activity demand, glucose stability, appetite pressure, prior exposure, and recovery capacity all influence how the body interprets continued reduction in incoming energy.

The Adaptive Efficiency Mechanism describes this process: the system may become more efficient under repeated energy constraint, narrowing the gap that originally produced fat loss.

The mechanism has two sides.

The first side is repeated constraint. Incoming energy is lower, body mass may be lower, and deficit pressure persists across time. The system receives the same general signal repeatedly: availability has changed.

The second side is efficiency adjustment. Output may decline. Movement may become less spontaneous. Appetite pressure may increase.

Recovery may be prioritized differently. Energy allocation may shift. The original gap between intake and expenditure may narrow.

This mechanism does not describe damage. It describes adjustment.

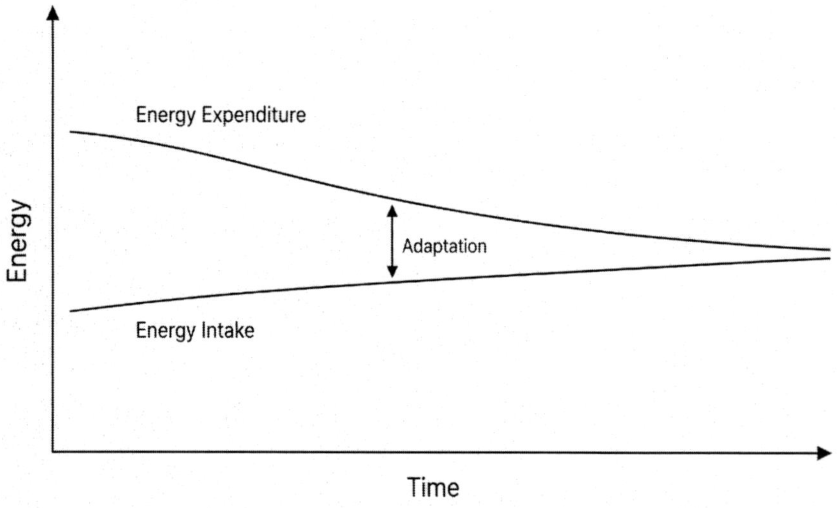

[Figure 11: Deficit Gap Narrowing Over Time]

The figure shows how the gap that initially supported fat loss can narrow as the system adapts. Energy intake begins below energy expenditure, creating a visible deficit gap. Over time, expenditure declines as body mass decreases, output changes, and efficiency adjustments occur. The space between intake and expenditure becomes smaller. The narrowing space represents adaptation.

The figure should not be interpreted as failure or permanent impairment. It shows that the body is adjusting to altered conditions. Lower body mass, reduced output, and efficiency changes can all reduce the original gap without implying that the system is broken.

This matters for fat loss stability because interpretation shapes response. If adaptation is interpreted as damage, the response often becomes panic, escalation, or overcorrection. The slowdown is treated as an emergency rather than information. More pressure may be added to a system already narrowing its tolerance for constraint.

If adaptation is understood as system adjustment, slower progress can be interpreted more accurately. The system has changed because the conditions have changed. The same input no longer produces the same output because the body has reorganized around sustained energy reduction.

This does not make adaptation a problem to fear. It makes adaptation a process to understand.

Fat loss stability depends not only on initiating reserve reduction, but on understanding how the system changes as reserve reduction continues. The body is not static during fat loss. It is responding, conserving, reallocating, and narrowing or widening its stability margins as conditions persist.

Chapter 12 moves into compensation, the next layer of this response. Adaptation describes internal adjustment under repeated constraint. Compensation describes the pressures that push appetite, behavior, output, and recovery back toward prior patterns.

Adaptation is not the failure of fat loss.

It is part of the regulation that determines whether fat loss remains stable over time.

Compensation: The System Pushes Back

Chapter 11 explained adaptation as internal system adjustment under repeated energy constraint. When reduced incoming energy persists, the body does not remain in the same state indefinitely. Energy output may decline. Movement may become less spontaneous. Efficiency may increase. Appetite pressure may rise. Recovery may become more difficult to support. The original gap between incoming energy and outgoing energy can narrow because the system has adjusted around the conditions it has been experiencing.

Compensation is the next layer of that response.

Adaptation describes changes in the system's operating state. Compensation describes the pressure that can emerge from those changes and push appetite, behavior, movement, output, and energy-seeking patterns back toward prior stability. The two processes overlap, but they are not identical. Adaptation changes how the system operates under constraint. Compensation changes the pressure surrounding behavior and output as the system attempts to restore availability or reduce expenditure.

This distinction matters because compensation is often misread as personal failure. Hunger becomes interpreted as weakness. Cravings become interpreted as lack of control. Reduced movement becomes interpreted as laziness. Lower output becomes interpreted as poor effort. Food focus becomes interpreted as obsession or inconsistency. These interpretations collapse regulatory pressure into character judgment.

From a systems perspective, compensation is not a moral event. It is a response to reduced availability.

When the system senses lower incoming energy, declining reserve availability, greater recovery burden, or narrowing stability margins, it may increase signals and behaviors that restore availability or conserve output. This does not mean fat loss is impossible. It means the system is producing return pressure. The direction of that pressure is toward a familiar range of intake, movement, energy availability, and functional stability.

Hunger is one of the most direct forms of compensation. As reduced energy availability persists, hunger may become more frequent, more urgent, or harder to background. It may appear earlier than expected, return sooner after eating, or feel more insistent during periods that previously felt stable. Hunger is not merely an idea or preference. It is a regulatory signal shaped by energy availability, sleep quality, stress load, glucose behavior, prior intake, recovery demand, and hormonal coordination.

In the context of fat loss, hunger can become part of the system's push toward restored availability. The body is detecting a changed energy environment and increasing the signal that encourages energy acquisition. This does not make hunger irrational. It makes hunger informative. It reflects the system's interpretation of constraint.

Food focus can develop alongside hunger, but it is not the same thing. Food focus is the increased mental prominence of eating, meals, snacks, convenience, portions, timing, or future food opportunities. When energy availability declines, attention may begin to narrow around energy acquisition. Food becomes easier to notice, harder to ignore, and more mentally available.

This should not be framed as weakness or obsession. Attention is part of regulation. A system perceiving reduced availability may allocate more cognitive priority toward food because food is the route through which availability can be restored. The mind becomes more attentive to energy opportunities when the body's regulatory environment is signaling constraint.

Cravings represent another form of compensation. They can intensify when the system seeks rapid, dense, familiar, or rewarding energy sources. Cravings are often moralized because they are attached to specific foods or eating patterns, but the underlying pressure is broader. The system may become more responsive to foods that offer quick availability, high reward, or strong sensory reinforcement when energy availability feels limited.

Cravings may become more prominent when sleep is disrupted, stress load is elevated, glucose is volatile, or prior restriction has increased urgency around food. In those conditions, the pressure is not only about preference. It is about signal intensity, reward sensitivity, and the system's attempt to restore availability efficiently.

Compensation also occurs through the output side of the system.

Energy output may decline in ways that are subtle enough to avoid notice. Spontaneous movement may decrease. Fidgeting may fade. Walking pace may slow. Posture may require less active muscular effort. Tasks may be delayed. Extra movement may feel less appealing. Physical effort may feel more costly than it did earlier. These changes may not appear as deliberate choices. They can emerge as the body reduces non-essential output under sustained energy constraint.

This connects to the adaptive efficiency mechanism from Chapter 11, but the emphasis here is slightly different. Adaptation describes the internal shift toward greater efficiency and lower expenditure. Compensation describes how that shift creates pressure in behavior and output. The body may conserve energy by making movement less automatic, less frequent, or less forceful. That conservation pushes the storage–release balance back toward prior stability by narrowing release-and-use pressure.

Fatigue can amplify this output compensation. When available energy, recovery capacity, and output demands become harder to coordinate, fatigue may rise. The system may become less tolerant of unnecessary effort, prolonged stress, extra movement, demanding tasks, or extended concentration. Ordinary activities may feel heavier. Recovery may take longer. The threshold for initiating effort may rise.

Fatigue is not always a simple lack of energy in the colloquial sense. It can be a regulatory signal that changes behavior before the system becomes more destabilized. By making effort feel more expensive, fatigue can reduce total output without requiring a conscious decision to reduce expenditure.

Lower tolerance belongs to the same pattern. The system may become less tolerant of skipped recovery, extra workload, intense activity, long gaps in energy availability, or repeated stress exposure. What was previously manageable may begin to feel harder under sustained constraint because the stability margin has narrowed. The same task may now require more recovery relative to available energy.

Movement decline should be understood carefully within this framework. Lower movement does not mean the person has become lazy. It can reflect energy conservation. When reduced availability persists, the body may lower non-essential output to preserve continuity. Deliberate activity may continue, but total daily movement can still decline through changes in posture, pacing, initiation, rest intervals, and spontaneous behavior.

This is one reason compensation can be difficult to detect. The person may believe the original structure is unchanged because the visible plan still looks the same. Yet the body may be producing less background movement, lower intensity, greater fatigue, stronger food focus, and more frequent appetite signals. The structure appears stable while the system's pressure environment has changed.

Compensation has two major directions.

The first direction is increased intake pressure. Hunger, cravings, food focus, eating urgency, reward sensitivity, and attention to food all increase the likelihood that energy intake will move back toward prior availability. This does not require dramatic overeating. It may appear as small additions, larger portions, more frequent eating, stronger pull toward convenience, or increased mental effort around food decisions.

The second direction is reduced output pressure. Lower spontaneous movement, reduced task intensity, fatigue, conservation, lower effort tolerance, and less frequent initiation of activity all reduce release-and-use pressure. Energy expenditure may decline not because of a deliberate decision to stop moving, but because the system is regulating around constraint.

These two directions affect fat loss stability from opposite sides of the same balance. Increased intake pressure can raise storage pressure. Reduced output can narrow release-and-use pressure. Together, they can reduce the gap that originally supported fat loss.

The important feature of compensation is that it may appear gradually. It may not feel like a dramatic physiological event. It may look like smaller portions becoming harder to maintain. Food decisions may become more mentally expensive. Movement may become easier to delay. Workouts may become less energetic. Ordinary tasks may feel heavier. Recovery may take longer. Sleep may become more fragile. The person may feel more drawn toward rest, convenience, or familiar energy sources.

Because these shifts can look ordinary, they are often misread as inconsistency. But from a systems perspective, they are predictable forms of pressure around reduced availability.

The system often pushes toward prior stability. Prior intake, prior body mass, prior appetite rhythm, prior movement output, and prior energy availability may represent a familiar operating state. When fat loss creates sustained deviation from that state, compensation can emerge as return pressure.

Return pressure is not conscious intention. The body is not plotting against fat loss. It is using feedback, signals, conservation, and behavioral pressure to move toward conditions that previously preserved continuity.

Compensation is therefore better understood as regulation around a changing baseline than as resistance in the moral sense.

The Compensation Pressure Mechanism defines this chapter's central claim: reduced energy availability can increase signals and behaviors that push the system back toward prior stability.

The mechanism has two sides.

The first side is reduced availability pressure. Incoming energy is lower, reserve access may become more constrained over time, recovery capacity may narrow, deficit pressure may persist, and adaptation may reduce the original energy gap. The system is operating under repeated constraint.

The second side is return pressure. Hunger rises. Cravings intensify. Food focus increases. Output declines. Movement becomes less spontaneous. Fatigue increases. Behavior drifts toward energy acquisition or conservation. Storage pressure may return as intake pressure rises or output falls.

Compensation does not mean fat loss cannot continue. It means the system is producing pressures that influence whether fat loss remains stable over time.

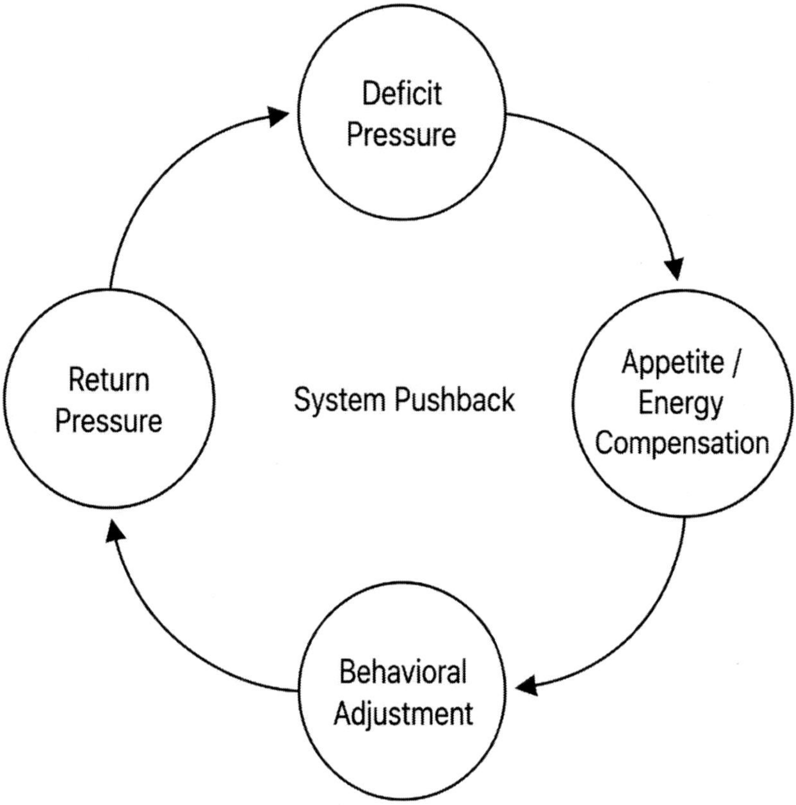

[Figure 12: Deficit → Compensation → Return Pressure]

The figure shows compensation as a loop rather than a single reaction. Deficit pressure increases appetite and energy compensation. Those pressures influence behavior and output. Behavioral adjustment creates return pressure toward prior stability. The center label, system pushback, describes regulation around reduced availability rather than failure.

This loop helps explain why fat loss can slow even when the original structure appears unchanged. The apparent plan may remain similar while appetite pressure rises, food focus increases, movement declines, fatigue accumulates, and output narrows. The system has not necessarily abandoned the process. It is regulating around constraint.

This also explains why a person can begin with stable effort and later experience stronger hunger, greater food attention, reduced movement, or declining output without making a conscious decision to change. Compensation can emerge gradually enough that it feels like normal variation until its cumulative effect becomes visible.

Chapter 13 will focus more directly on appetite pressure, one of the most important interfaces between internal regulation and eating behavior. Hunger, cravings, urgency, and food focus are not peripheral to fat loss stability. They are central signals through which the system communicates reduced availability and pushes toward restoration.

Compensation is not character failure. It is regulatory pressure that can push the system back toward prior stability unless the broader system remains coordinated enough to continue.

Appetite Pressure and Fat Loss Instability

Chapter 12 explained compensation as return pressure under reduced energy availability. Compensation can emerge through increased intake pressure, reduced output pressure, or both. Hunger may intensify. Food focus may increase. Movement may decline. Fatigue may rise. These responses are not separate from regulation. They are part of the system's attempt to preserve continuity under changing energy conditions.

Appetite pressure belongs primarily to the intake side of compensation, but its effects extend beyond eating alone. Appetite influences focus, urgency, reward sensitivity, timing pressure, decision friction, and behavioral drift. It is one of the main ways internal regulation becomes behaviorally visible.

This is why appetite occupies such a central role in fat loss stability. Appetite is not merely a preference system. It is the behavioral interface of energy regulation. Internal conditions become felt through appetite as hunger, cravings, fullness, satiety, food focus, urgency, eating motivation, and perceived energy need. Appetite translates physiology into behaviorally relevant signals.

When energy availability changes, appetite pressure often changes with it.

Reduced intake, prolonged deficit pressure, changing stored reserves, elevated stress load, poor sleep, unstable glucose behavior, inadequate recovery, repeated prior restriction, and high activity demand can all influence appetite signaling. These variables do not produce identical responses in every person or every condition, but they shape the environment in which hunger and satiety are interpreted.

Hunger is one of the clearest expressions of this process. Hunger is not simply desire for food, and it is not adequately explained as lack of discipline. Hunger is a regulatory signal linked to perceived energy availability. When the system interprets incoming energy or reserve availability as insufficient relative to demand, hunger pressure may increase.

That increase may appear through frequency, intensity, persistence, or urgency. Hunger may arrive sooner after eating. It may feel more difficult to ignore. It may interrupt concentration more often. The pressure associated with hunger may become more behaviorally influential as reduced availability persists.

Hunger should not be framed as irrational, but it also should not be interpreted as an unquestionable command. From a systems perspective, hunger is information. It reflects the body's attempt to communicate changing availability conditions through behavioral pressure.

Satiety belongs to the same regulatory framework. Satiety is not merely stomach fullness. It is the broader sense of satisfaction and reduced eating drive that follows intake. Under stable conditions, satiety may remain relatively durable across time. Meals may create a period of reduced urgency before hunger gradually returns.

Under sustained energy constraint, satiety durability may change.

Meals may feel less satisfying than they previously did. Fullness may fade more quickly. The interval between eating and renewed hunger may shorten. A person may finish eating while still feeling mentally attentive to food. These shifts can occur even when the visible structure remains similar because the system is interpreting energy availability differently.

This distinction matters because satiety loss is often misread behaviorally instead of regulatorily. If meals no longer feel as satisfying under reduced availability, the experience may appear inconsistent or emotionally confusing. Yet from a systems perspective, the body is adjusting appetite signaling relative to changing energy conditions.

Cravings develop within this same environment. Cravings can intensify when the system becomes more responsive to rapid, dense, familiar, or highly rewarding energy sources. Cravings are often moralized because they are associated with specific foods, but the deeper issue is reward sensitivity under altered availability conditions.

The system may increase responsiveness to foods associated with quick energy acquisition when energy pressure rises. This does not require framing certain foods as "bad" or "addictive" in simplistic terms. The more useful interpretation is that reward salience changes under conditions of reduced availability, elevated stress, unstable glucose, poor recovery, or repeated restriction exposure.

Cravings therefore represent signal pressure within a changed regulatory environment. Stress can intensify them. Sleep disruption can intensify them. Glucose volatility can intensify them. Repeated cycles of restriction and compensation can intensify them. Appetite pressure becomes more behaviorally forceful when multiple instability layers overlap.

Food focus represents another expression of appetite compensation. Food focus is the mental prominence of eating-related thought. Attention may narrow around meals, portions, timing, snacks, convenience, future eating opportunities, or available food cues. Food may occupy more cognitive space than it did under more stable energy conditions.

This should not automatically be interpreted as pathology. The mind becoming more attentive to energy acquisition under reduced availability is understandable within a regulatory framework. Cognitive attention shifts toward biologically relevant needs. When energy pressure rises, food-related information can become more behaviorally important.

Food urgency develops when appetite pressure intensifies further. Urgency is the felt pressure that eating needs to happen soon, or that delaying a food response feels increasingly difficult. Hunger, fatigue, glucose volatility, stress load, and narrowed recovery capacity can converge into stronger urgency signals.

Urgency should not be interpreted as weakness or lack of control. It is better understood as increased signal intensity. The system is raising behavioral pressure around energy acquisition because availability feels increasingly constrained relative to demand.

This becomes especially important when appetite pressure begins changing behavior gradually rather than dramatically.

Compensation rarely appears as a single catastrophic event. More often, it develops through accumulation. Portions become slightly larger. Delays become harder to tolerate. Snacking becomes more frequent. Evening intake pressure rises. Convenience foods become more appealing. Reward sensitivity increases. Food decisions require more mental effort. The structure that initially felt relatively stable becomes progressively more difficult to maintain.

These changes may appear small in isolation. Their significance emerges through repetition across time.

This is one reason appetite pressure is frequently misunderstood. The visible structure may appear mostly unchanged while internal behavioral pressure increases steadily. A person may believe they are failing to maintain consistency when, in reality, the system is generating stronger intake-oriented signals under reduced availability conditions.

Appetite pressure therefore influences the storage–release balance directly.

When appetite pressure rises, intake pressure often rises with it. Increased intake pressure can narrow the deficit signal, reduce release-and-use pressure, or increase storage pressure across time. Appetite does not need to completely reverse fat loss in order to alter the environment supporting it. Even modest increases in eating frequency, portion size, reward responsiveness, or energy-seeking behavior can gradually shift the balance.

The important point is not that appetite "ruins" fat loss. The more accurate systems interpretation is that appetite changes the conditions fat loss depends on.

Fat loss stability depends partly on whether appetite signals remain within a tolerable range relative to the system's capacity. "Tolerable" here should not be interpreted morally or behaviorally. It refers to whether appetite pressure remains within a range the broader system can absorb without escalating compensation strongly enough to destabilize continuity.

When appetite pressure remains relatively tolerable, reduced availability may coexist with manageable hunger, stable satiety, and relatively consistent behavior. When appetite pressure rises beyond that tolerance range, compensation becomes more likely. Hunger may intensify further. Cravings may become more intrusive. Food urgency may rise. Behavioral drift may accumulate. Intake pressure may increasingly overpower the conditions supporting release-and-use pressure.

This does not mean fat loss becomes impossible. It means the regulatory environment is becoming more compensatory.

The Appetite Compensation Mechanism defines this process clearly: changing energy availability can increase appetite pressure until behavior begins to compensate.

The mechanism has two sides.

The first side is energy availability change. Reduced intake, changing stored reserves, elevated demand, unstable glucose behavior, poor recovery, stress load, and prior restriction all contribute to the perception of changing availability. The system is interpreting a shift in energy conditions.

The second side is appetite pressure response. Hunger intensifies. Cravings become more prominent. Satiety durability weakens. Food focus increases. Urgency rises. Reward sensitivity becomes stronger. Behavior begins drifting toward restored availability.

Appetite pressure becomes destabilizing when it shifts behavior strongly enough to alter the storage–release balance. The destabilization is not caused by weakness. It emerges because regulatory pressure is influencing intake patterns, eating behavior, and energy acquisition priorities.

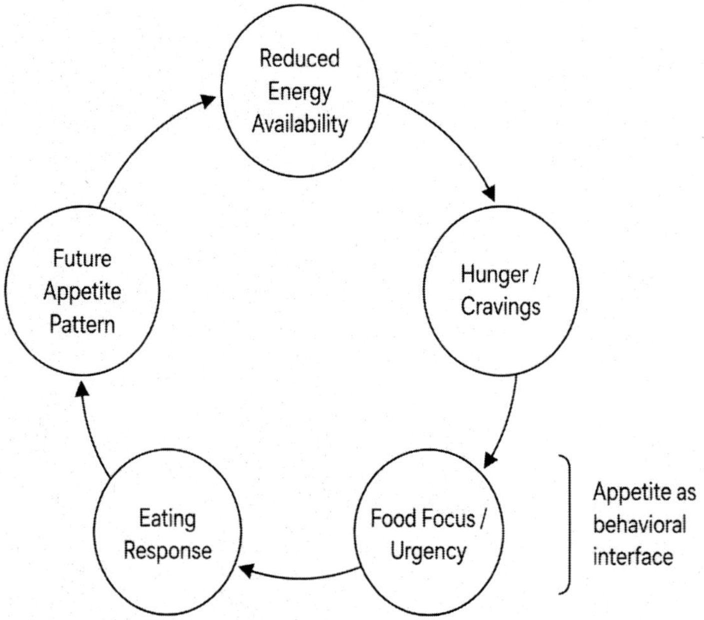

[Figure 13: Appetite Pressure Loop]

The figure presents appetite pressure as a loop rather than a single sensation. Reduced energy availability increases hunger and cravings. Hunger and cravings increase food focus and urgency. Food focus and urgency influence eating response. Eating responses shape future appetite patterns and perceived availability conditions, feeding back into the beginning of the cycle.

The loop can remain relatively stable or become increasingly compensatory depending on system conditions. Stable sleep, manageable stress, coherent recovery, and relatively stable glucose behavior may reduce the amplification of appetite pressure. Poor sleep, elevated stress, repeated restriction, unstable glucose, and prolonged deficit pressure may intensify the loop and increase behavioral compensation.

This loop helps explain why appetite changes often appear gradually during fat loss attempts. A person may begin with relatively stable structure and later experience stronger hunger, reduced satiety durability, more food focus, or greater urgency without consciously deciding to abandon the process. The system is communicating changing availability conditions through appetite.

The behavioral relevance of appetite is what makes it such an important interface in fat loss stability. Appetite sits at the boundary between internal regulation and outward behavior. Signals related to availability, recovery, stress, and stored energy become behaviorally influential through appetite pressure.

This is also why appetite cannot be reduced to simple willpower language. Appetite operates inside a layered regulatory environment shaped by sleep quality, stress exposure, glucose behavior, recovery burden, prior energy availability, hormonal coordination, reward sensitivity, and ongoing deficit pressure. Treating appetite entirely as choice removes the regulatory system from view.

At the same time, appetite should not be framed fatalistically. Appetite pressure is influential, but it is not proof that fat loss cannot occur. The more precise interpretation is that appetite becomes one of the major pressures determining whether reduced availability remains stable or becomes increasingly compensatory across time.

Chapter 14 will examine one of the major amplifiers of appetite instability: blood sugar and glucose volatility. Appetite pressure is one behavioral surface of energy regulation. Glucose behavior influences hunger intensity, fatigue, cravings, urgency, reward sensitivity, and perceived energy availability. Variability in glucose regulation can therefore intensify appetite compensation even when external structure appears relatively consistent.

Appetite pressure is not a failure of control. It is the behavioral surface of energy regulation, and it can determine whether fat loss remains stable or becomes increasingly compensatory over time.

Blood Sugar, Glucose Volatility, and Fat Loss

Chapter 13 explained appetite pressure as the behavioral surface of energy regulation. Hunger, cravings, satiety loss, food focus, urgency, and eating motivation are not separate from physiology. They are ways the system communicates changing energy conditions through behaviorally relevant signals. Appetite pressure can intensify when the body interprets reduced or unstable availability, particularly under prolonged deficit pressure, elevated stress load, inadequate recovery, or changing stored reserves.

Chapter 14 focuses on one condition that can amplify that pressure: glucose volatility.

Blood sugar is one of the most visible and immediately felt signals in the metabolic system. Glucose behavior influences perceived energy availability, hunger intensity, fatigue, cravings, urgency, concentration, and willingness to sustain effort. Because glucose is so visible and experiential, it is often given excessive explanatory power. Some frameworks treat blood sugar as the master variable governing fat loss. Others dismiss it entirely. Both interpretations flatten the system.

Glucose matters, but it matters within a larger regulatory environment.

The significance of glucose behavior in fat loss stability is not that blood sugar directly determines whether stored reserves decline. The more precise issue is that unstable glucose patterns can destabilize the conditions fat loss depends on. Volatility in perceived energy availability can intensify compensation pressure through hunger, fatigue, cravings, urgency, reactive eating pressure, and reduced output tolerance.

Glucose volatility refers to unstable rises and falls in glucose availability across time. These fluctuations alter how energy availability is perceived and regulated. The issue is not whether glucose rises at all. Glucose movement is part of normal physiology. The issue is the stability, magnitude, frequency, and recovery pattern of those fluctuations across changing conditions.

From a systems perspective, glucose behavior functions partly as an availability signal. When glucose availability appears stable and predictable, energy conditions may feel relatively coherent. When glucose availability becomes more volatile, the system may interpret availability as less stable, even if total energy intake across time remains similar.

This distinction is important because glucose volatility influences pressure rather than acting as a direct command.

Stable glucose does not guarantee fat loss. A person can experience relatively stable glucose patterns while remaining in a storage-supportive environment overall. Likewise, unstable glucose does not make fat loss impossible. Stored reserves can still decline under volatile conditions. The relevant point is narrower and more useful: glucose volatility can make the conditions supporting fat loss more difficult to sustain.

The destabilizing effect occurs largely through compensation pressure.

Hunger is one of the clearest pathways through which this happens. When glucose availability fluctuates sharply, hunger may become more urgent, more frequent, or less predictable. Falling availability signals may increase intake pressure, particularly when reduced incoming energy, elevated stress, unstable recovery, or prior restriction are already present.

The system is not responding only to objective energy quantity. It is also responding to perceived availability stability. Rapid changes in perceived availability can intensify pressure around eating because the body is attempting to restore more stable conditions.

This can make hunger feel more behaviorally forceful. A person may experience stronger urgency between meals, shorter satiety intervals, or more abrupt transitions from stable energy to perceived depletion. Hunger may feel less gradual and more reactive.

These experiences are often interpreted psychologically or morally, especially when they emerge suddenly. Yet glucose volatility provides one possible systems explanation for why appetite pressure may intensify even when visible structure appears relatively similar.

Fatigue develops through a related pathway.

Glucose volatility can contribute to perceived energy instability. Energy may feel less predictable across the day. Concentration may become less steady. Fatigue may emerge more abruptly. Motivation for effort may fluctuate more sharply. These experiences are not produced by glucose alone, but unstable glucose behavior can amplify them.

The relevant issue is not simply "low energy." The more accurate interpretation is inconsistent perceived availability.

When the system alternates between periods of higher and lower perceived glucose availability, energy perception itself may become unstable. Fatigue can therefore become part of the compensation environment. The body may reduce willingness to sustain effort, initiate movement, tolerate stress, or maintain output when perceived availability becomes less reliable.

This matters because fatigue influences both the intake side and output side of the storage–release balance.

On the intake side, fatigue may increase reward-seeking behavior, convenience orientation, and urgency around rapid availability. On the output side, fatigue may reduce spontaneous movement, willingness to initiate effort, posture energy, task persistence, or physical output across time.

These shifts do not require conscious decisions. Much of the compensation associated with energy instability occurs subtly through altered behavioral pressure.

Cravings represent another major pathway through which glucose volatility can destabilize the fat-loss environment.

When perceived availability becomes unstable, the system may become more responsive to rapid or familiar energy sources. Reward sensitivity may increase when falling availability signals coincide with fatigue, stress load, or appetite pressure. Cravings therefore emerge partly through the interaction between energy instability and reward-oriented compensation.

This should not be moralized into "good" versus "bad" foods. The deeper issue is rapid-availability seeking under unstable energy conditions.

The body may become more attentive to foods associated with quick energy acquisition when urgency rises. Cravings become more behaviorally forceful not because the person lacks discipline, but because the system is increasing reward salience around restoring perceived availability.

Stress, poor sleep, prior restriction exposure, and prolonged deficit pressure can intensify this process further. Glucose volatility rarely operates in isolation. It interacts with the broader regulatory environment already developed throughout the book.

Urgency becomes especially important within this interaction.

Glucose volatility can make eating feel increasingly time-sensitive. Hunger may feel more abrupt. Fatigue may appear more suddenly. Irritability, shakiness, reduced concentration, or perceived depletion may increase the felt pressure to respond quickly to food-related signals.

Urgency should not be interpreted as weakness or overreaction. It is better understood as signal intensity.

The more unstable availability feels, the more rapidly the system may push toward restoration behavior. This is particularly relevant during periods of reduced intake, elevated stress, inadequate recovery, or prolonged compensation pressure. The overlap between appetite instability and glucose volatility can amplify the behavioral pull toward eating.

Reactive eating pressure emerges when hunger, cravings, fatigue, and urgency begin converging into a stronger compensation environment.

Reactive eating does not mean irrational eating. It means eating behavior becomes increasingly shaped by short-term pressure signals rather than stable availability conditions. Eating may become more impulsive, more convenience-oriented, more reward-sensitive, or more urgency-driven when perceived availability feels unstable.

This can happen gradually rather than dramatically.

A person may begin paying more attention to quick energy sources. Delays between meals may feel harder to tolerate. Evening intake pressure may rise after periods of fatigue or energy instability. Eating decisions may become more reactive under stress or exhaustion. These shifts often appear ordinary, which is why they are frequently misread as inconsistency or lack of commitment rather than compensation pressure.

Reactive eating pressure matters because it influences the storage–release balance developed in earlier chapters.

When intake pressure rises repeatedly under unstable energy conditions, storage pressure may increase or release-and-use pressure may become less stable. The deficit signal may narrow. Compensation may intensify. Eating patterns may become less predictable or more reward-responsive.

The issue is not that one reactive eating episode eliminates fat loss. The larger issue is that repeated instability can alter the long-term environment supporting release and use across time.

Glucose volatility therefore influences fat loss indirectly through pressure modulation rather than direct control.

This distinction protects against two oversimplifications.

The first oversimplification treats glucose stability as a guaranteed solution. The second treats glucose behavior as irrelevant. A systems interpretation avoids both extremes.

Stable glucose may reduce one layer of appetite and energy volatility, but fat loss still depends on the broader relationship between storage pressure and release-and-use pressure. Access, mobilization, utilization, recovery capacity, stress load, demand, hormonal coordination, and appetite regulation all remain relevant.

At the same time, unstable glucose behavior can increase compensation pressure strongly enough to destabilize continuity even when the broader structure initially appears workable.

This interaction becomes especially important under stress and poor recovery conditions.

Sleep disruption can amplify glucose instability while simultaneously increasing appetite pressure and reducing recovery capacity. Stress signaling can alter glucose availability patterns while increasing reward sensitivity and urgency. Reduced recovery may increase fatigue while lowering tolerance for instability.

The result is not simply "higher blood sugar" or "lower blood sugar." The result is a less predictable availability environment.

When energy availability feels inconsistent, compensation pressure may rise across multiple layers simultaneously. Hunger increases. Fatigue becomes more prominent. Cravings intensify. Output tolerance declines. Urgency becomes more behaviorally influential. The system begins pushing harder toward restored availability and reduced strain.

Glucose volatility also influences the output side of regulation.

Energy instability may reduce willingness to sustain effort, initiate movement, maintain posture energy, or tolerate prolonged activity. Training drive may feel less stable. Task initiation may become more difficult. Movement may become more conservative or inconsistent.

This matters because fat loss stability depends partly on continuity of release-and-use pressure. If energy instability reduces movement or output tolerance across time, the conditions supporting release-and-use pressure may narrow.

The interaction between intake compensation and output compensation becomes especially important here.

Fatigue increases eating pressure while simultaneously reducing output tolerance. Hunger increases urgency while movement becomes more difficult to sustain. Reward sensitivity rises while recovery capacity narrows. Glucose volatility can therefore intensify compensation from both directions at once.

The Glucose Compensation Mechanism defines this process clearly: glucose volatility can increase eating pressure, energy instability, and perceived urgency.

The mechanism has two sides.

The first side is glucose volatility itself. Availability signals become less stable across time. Glucose rises and falls more sharply or less predictably. Energy perception becomes more inconsistent. The system experiences greater instability in perceived availability.

The second side is compensatory pressure. Hunger rises. Fatigue becomes more prominent. Cravings intensify. Urgency increases. Reactive eating pressure strengthens. Output tolerance declines. Behavior becomes less stable under rising compensation pressure.

The mechanism does not mean glucose volatility directly controls fat loss. Fat loss is not reducible to one variable. The more precise interpretation is that glucose volatility can destabilize the pressure environment fat loss depends on.

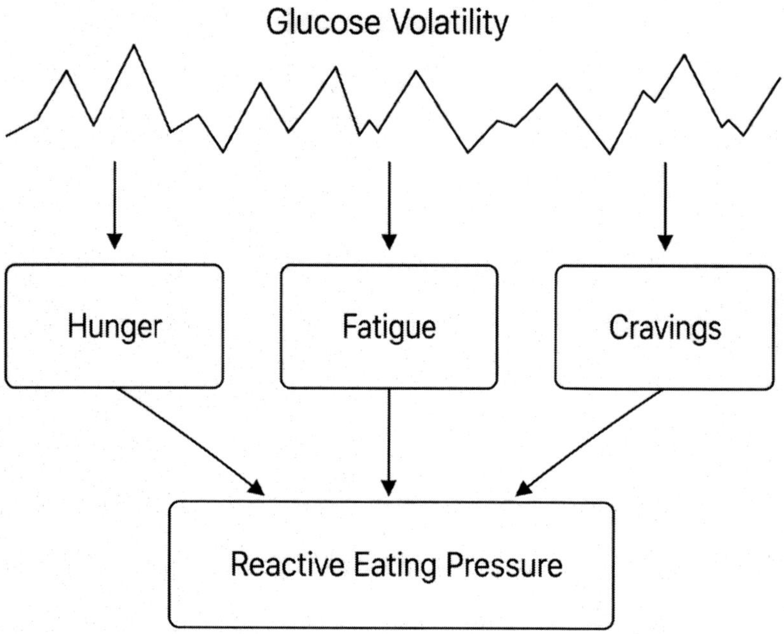

[Figure 14: Glucose Volatility → Hunger/Energy Compensation]

The figure illustrates this relationship visually. Glucose volatility appears at the top as a jagged availability signal moving across time. Downward arrows connect that instability to hunger, fatigue, and cravings. Those pressures then converge into reactive eating pressure.

The figure should not be interpreted as claiming glucose is the sole cause of hunger, fatigue, or cravings. Appetite pressure, stress load, recovery status, sleep quality, hormonal coordination, and stored-energy conditions all remain relevant. The figure instead isolates one important pathway: unstable energy availability can amplify compensation pressure through multiple overlapping signals.

This matters because glucose volatility is often interpreted behaviorally rather than regulatorily.

A person may experience sudden hunger, fatigue, cravings, irritability, or urgency and conclude that they are inconsistent, unmotivated, or unable to sustain fat loss structure. A systems interpretation offers a different explanation. Signal instability may be increasing the pressure environment surrounding eating and output behavior.

This does not remove personal agency, but it changes interpretation. The issue is not moral failure. The issue is that unstable availability signals can increase compensation pressure strongly enough to alter behavior across time.

The broader significance of this chapter is therefore stability, not perfection.

The goal is not to eliminate every glucose fluctuation. Glucose behavior is inherently dynamic because metabolism itself is dynamic. The more relevant issue is whether volatility becomes strong enough to amplify hunger, fatigue, cravings, urgency, and reactive compensation beyond the system's ability to maintain continuity comfortably.

Chapter 15 will extend this discussion into energy demand and daily function. Appetite pressure and glucose volatility influence the intake side and perceived energy side of the system. The next chapter examines the output side more directly: how movement, activity demand, daily function, and energy expenditure interact with stored-energy use.

Glucose stability does not produce fat loss by itself. But glucose volatility can make fat loss less stable by increasing hunger, fatigue, cravings, urgency, and reactive compensation pressure across time.

Energy Demand and Daily Function

Chapter 14 examined glucose volatility as one way the fat-loss environment can become less stable. Unstable glucose patterns can amplify hunger, fatigue, cravings, urgency, and reactive eating pressure while reducing output tolerance. Those effects often appear on the intake side of the system, where perceived energy instability increases appetite pressure and makes eating behavior more reactive. But glucose volatility can also influence the output side by changing fatigue, effort tolerance, movement, and the willingness to sustain daily function.

Chapter 15 shifts more directly toward that output side.

Fat loss depends partly on demand because released energy needs a destination. Stored energy must become accessible, mobilized, circulated, and used. Demand helps create the conditions in which released energy becomes useful rather than merely available. Without sufficient demand, mobilized energy has less reason to be used by tissues in a way that contributes to meaningful stored-reserve reduction.

This does not mean demand should be reduced to formal exercise. Exercise is visible, labeled, measurable, and easy to isolate. Because of that visibility, it often receives more explanatory power than it can carry by itself. A workout can be identified, counted, timed, and remembered. Daily output is more diffuse. It is spread across walking, standing, posture, task effort, fidgeting, work tolerance, household movement, training quality, stress regulation, and ordinary function.

Energy Stability frames daily energy as functional output across time. In that same sense, demand is not a single event. It is the body's continuing requirement for energy to move, think, work, recover, regulate temperature, maintain posture, respond to stress, and perform ordinary responsibilities. Fat loss occurs inside that broader daily-function environment, not only inside the visible window of planned activity.

Structured exercise can increase demand. It can support glucose use, preserve function, contribute to movement capacity, and create a context in which released energy becomes relevant. But it should not be interpreted as a direct fat-loss transaction. Exercise is not a payment for food, a punishment for intake, or a mechanical guarantee that stored fat will decline. It is one contributor to the demand side of the system.

The body does not separate demand into culturally labeled categories. It responds to total output, recovery demand, tissue work, stress load, and available energy. A planned workout may be one visible expression of demand, but it exists alongside many smaller forms of energy use that accumulate across the day.

Walking and ordinary movement are part of that accumulation. Movement between activities, errands, standing, household tasks, transitions, carrying objects, and shifting from one place to another all contribute to the daily energy environment. These forms of output may not feel like exercise because they are embedded in ordinary function. Yet they still require energy, coordination, and tissue work.

Posture and physical tone also contribute. Sitting upright, standing, maintaining balance, moving efficiently, carrying the body through space, and remaining physically engaged throughout the day all require background muscular activity. When energy availability narrows or fatigue rises, posture and tone may decline subtly. A person may sit more heavily, move less frequently, stand for shorter periods, or conserve physical engagement without consciously deciding to reduce output.

Fidgeting and spontaneous movement are even less visible. Shifting position, gesturing, pacing, changing posture, tapping, rising from a chair, or making small non-deliberate movements can all decline when the system begins conserving energy. These movements are minor individually, but they reflect the body's background output state. Under energy constraint, small forms of movement can fade without being noticed.

Task effort and work tolerance extend the demand model beyond physical movement alone. Cognitive work, sustained attention, decision-making, emotional regulation, and task persistence all require energy coordination. The brain is not separate from the energy system. When fatigue rises or perceived availability becomes unstable, effort can feel more expensive. Concentration may become harder to sustain. Tasks may be delayed. Decision-making may feel heavier. Output can decline even when no formal exercise variable has changed.

Training output has its own hidden variability. A person may maintain the same workout schedule while the actual output changes. Intensity may decline. Volume may drift downward. Rest periods may increase. Movement quality may reduce. Enthusiasm may fall. Recovery may take longer. The visible plan remains the same, but the physiological demand created by the session is no longer identical.

This matters because fat loss interpretation often relies too heavily on visible structure. The calendar may still show the same workouts. The routine may appear unchanged. Yet hidden output may have shifted across training intensity, spontaneous movement, posture, task effort, and daily function.

General daily function ties these layers together. Daily function includes the ability to move, think, work, regulate stress, maintain routine, recover, and carry out ordinary responsibilities. Fat loss conditions are more stable when daily function remains intact because the system can maintain release-and-use pressure without excessive compensation. When daily function deteriorates, appetite pressure, fatigue, stress load, and output decline often rise together.

This is where demand connects directly to the adaptation and compensation chapters.

Under repeated energy constraint, adaptation may reduce output. The system may become more efficient, lower spontaneous movement, conserve effort, or narrow the energy gap that originally supported fat loss. Compensation may then appear as fatigue, lower movement, reduced effort tolerance, or increased appetite pressure. Demand stability protects against the loss of release-and-use pressure, but demand itself can become unstable when the system is under sustained constraint.

Hidden output decline is one of the most important expressions of this instability. It can appear as slower pacing, more sitting, reduced spontaneous movement, diminished posture energy, lower task intensity, reduced training drive, or shorter tolerance for activity. These changes can narrow release-and-use pressure even when the visible plan appears unchanged.

This is one reason fat loss can slow without an obvious change in behavior. The behavior being tracked may remain stable while the behavior not being tracked shifts quietly. Planned exercise may continue while total daily movement declines. Food structure may appear consistent while fatigue reduces output. Workouts may remain scheduled while training quality falls. The system may be conserving energy through channels that do not look like deliberate decisions.

Demand must be present because released energy requires use. If tissues do not require energy, mobilized fuel has less reason to contribute to stored-reserve reduction. Demand gives released energy direction. It connects access and mobilization to utilization.

Demand must also be tolerable. When demand exceeds recovery capacity, it can increase fatigue, appetite pressure, stress signaling, and compensation. A high-demand period may increase expenditure initially, but if it destabilizes recovery, later output may decline or intake pressure may rise. The system may preserve continuity by reducing movement, increasing hunger, or shifting energy allocation.

Demand must be sustainable because fat loss depends on patterns across time. A single high-demand moment does not replace stable daily function. Short bursts of output can be offset by later compensation if the system cannot recover from them. The goal in this chapter is not to elevate more demand as inherently better. The point is that demand supports fat loss most effectively when it remains present without overwhelming the system that must sustain it.

This is the Demand Stability Mechanism: stored energy is more likely to be used when energy demand remains present, tolerable, and sustainable.

The mechanism has three sides.

Present demand means tissues need energy, creating a destination for released fuel. Tolerable demand means the demand does not exceed recovery capacity so strongly that compensation rises faster than utilization. Sustainable demand means the demand can persist across time without collapsing output, increasing return pressure, or destabilizing daily function.

This mechanism does not mean more activity is always better. It means demand works best when it supports continued function.

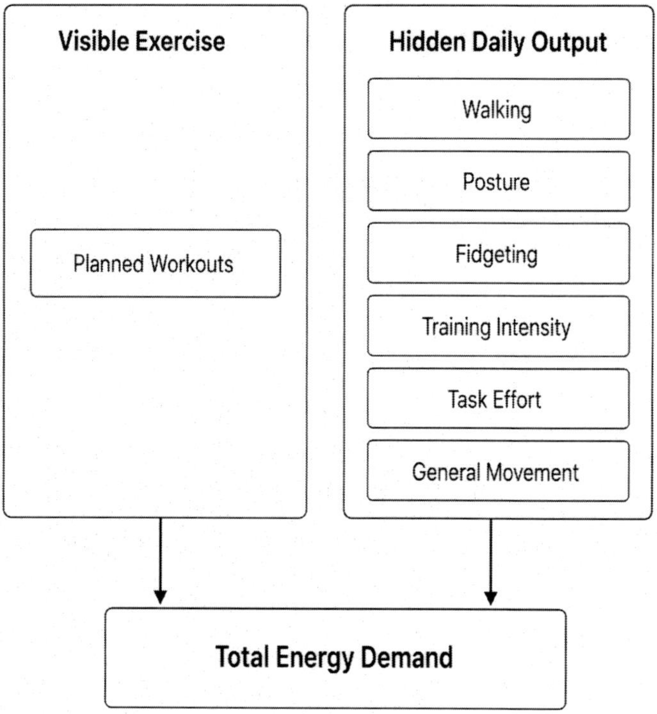

[Figure 15: Visible Exercise vs Hidden Daily Output]

The figure separates visible exercise from hidden daily output. Planned workouts appear in the visible exercise column because they are easy to identify and measure. Walking, posture, fidgeting, training intensity, task effort, and general movement appear in the hidden daily output column because they often change without being noticed. Both columns feed into total energy demand.

The figure prevents the assumption that unchanged workouts mean unchanged total output. A person may maintain the same visible exercise routine while hidden daily output declines. The formal structure remains visible, but the total demand environment shifts underneath it.

This distinction matters for fat loss interpretation. When fat loss slows, the visible plan may appear unchanged. Exercise may still be present. Food structure may still appear similar. But hidden variables may have shifted:

less spontaneous movement, lower training intensity, slower pacing, more fatigue, reduced task effort, poorer recovery, or diminished posture energy. These changes can narrow release-and-use pressure and contribute to a plateau.

The opposite error is also important. Demand that becomes too aggressive may increase compensation and reduce stability. If output is pushed beyond recovery capacity, appetite pressure may rise, fatigue may intensify, stress signaling may increase, and later movement may decline. In that case, more demand in one area can reduce total demand across time by destabilizing the system supporting it.

Both errors come from misunderstanding demand as simple exercise volume.

Demand is better understood as the total functional output of the system. It includes the visible and the hidden, the formal and the ordinary, the planned and the spontaneous. It changes with energy availability, glucose stability, sleep, stress, recovery, appetite pressure, adaptation, and daily responsibilities.

Chapter 16 will examine plateaus as system feedback. Plateaus often occur when the visible plan appears unchanged but underlying variables have shifted. Hidden output decline, demand changes, fatigue, recovery strain, water retention, intake drift, adaptation, stress load, and glucose volatility can all contribute to a stalled visible outcome.

Fat loss depends not on maximal demand, but on demand that remains present, tolerable, and sustainable enough for stored energy to keep moving toward use over time.

Plateaus as System Feedback

Chapter 15 explained that the visible structure of a fat-loss attempt can remain relatively stable while hidden output shifts quietly underneath it. A person may continue following the same apparent routine while daily movement declines, posture energy softens, task effort narrows, training quality decreases, or recovery strain rises. The visible plan can therefore remain unchanged while the underlying energy environment changes substantially. The same interpretive caution applies to visible fat-loss outcomes themselves. A plateau often appears as stalled change, but the visible stall does not automatically explain why it is occurring.

This distinction matters because plateaus are commonly interpreted as direct evidence of failure. Visible slowing is treated as proof that the system has stopped responding, that the process is no longer working, or that something inside the body has become resistant or damaged. The interpretation arrives quickly because the visible signal appears simple. Weight stops moving, measurements flatten, or outward changes become less obvious, and the mind immediately attempts to convert the observation into a complete explanation. But the observation and the explanation are not the same thing.

A plateau is best understood first as a visible event. It is a period in which visible change appears slower, less responsive, or harder to detect than expected. This may appear through body weight, waist measurements, clothing fit, mirror perception, or other outward markers used to judge progress across time. The key point is not the specific marker itself. The key point is that the plateau represents an observation of the visible signal becoming flatter or less clear.

That visible observation does not automatically reveal the underlying mechanism responsible for it. A plateau is not a diagnosis. It is not a final verdict about whether fat loss is still occurring underneath the visible surface. It is not automatic proof that stored energy reduction has stopped entirely. It is not automatic evidence that the system is broken, resistant, or no longer responsive. A plateau means the visible signal has become more difficult to interpret clearly.

The scale creates particular confusion because it compresses many variables into one number. Body weight is often treated as though it were a direct meter for fat mass, but body weight reflects far more than stored fat alone. Water distribution, glycogen status, digestive contents, sodium-related fluid behavior, inflammation-related fluid shifts, tissue repair, and other compartments all contribute to total weight at a given moment. The visible number therefore functions as a composite signal rather than as a direct reading of stored-energy change itself.

This distinction becomes increasingly important during periods of sustained fat loss because many of the same conditions that influence stored-energy reduction also influence fluid behavior, recovery demand, appetite pressure, and system stress. Visible weight may therefore flatten temporarily even while the broader system continues changing underneath.

Water retention is one of the most common reasons visible change becomes temporarily obscured. Fluid behavior is highly responsive to stress load, recovery burden, inflammation, sleep quality, training strain, sodium shifts, hormonal fluctuations, and glycogen status. When recovery demand rises or stress accumulates, fluid retention may increase even if stored fat is continuing to decline underneath. The visible outcome can therefore appear stalled despite ongoing changes within the storage–release system.

This creates interpretive confusion because water shifts occur more quickly than fat-mass changes. A relatively small change in fluid distribution can temporarily outweigh slower changes in stored energy. The scale may therefore appear flat, unchanged, or temporarily elevated during periods when stored reserves are still gradually declining underneath the visible signal.

Glycogen shifts add another layer of ambiguity because glycogen is stored alongside water. When glycogen stores rise, associated water retention rises with them. When glycogen stores fall, associated fluid may decrease as well. These shifts can produce visible movement in body weight that does not perfectly reflect changes in stored fat mass itself.

A replenishment phase may therefore temporarily increase visible weight even when fat accumulation has not increased at the same pace. A depletion phase may temporarily decrease visible weight without representing equivalent fat loss. Visible plateaus may similarly reflect glycogen-associated fluid behavior rather than a perfect mirror of stored-energy dynamics. The visible signal becomes harder to interpret because multiple compartments are moving simultaneously.

Digestive contents create another form of temporary masking that is often overlooked because it feels too ordinary to matter. Food volume, fluid intake, digestive timing, and material moving through the gastrointestinal system all contribute to body weight at a given time. This does not represent fat gain. It reflects the reality that body weight measures total mass, not stored fat in isolation.

The timing of meals, differences in food volume, variations in digestion, and changes in bowel movement patterns can therefore influence visible weight independently of fat-mass change. A person may interpret temporary stability as failure when the visible signal partly reflects ordinary digestive variation rather than a true stop in stored-energy reduction.

Inflammation and recovery-related fluid shifts further complicate interpretation because tissue repair itself alters fluid behavior. Training strain, accumulated fatigue, soreness, poor sleep, psychological stress, or elevated recovery demand may increase water retention associated with repair processes. A person may assume fat loss has stopped because the visible number no longer declines, while the body is simultaneously managing tissue recovery, inflammation signaling, and fluid redistribution underneath the surface.

The same confusion appears in periods of higher stress load. Stress affects far more than emotional state alone. It can influence water retention, appetite pressure, glucose behavior, recovery quality, perceived urgency, sleep stability, and output tolerance simultaneously. This does not mean stress alone explains every plateau, nor does it mean stress acts as a magical barrier preventing fat loss. It means stress changes the broader regulatory environment in ways that can either slow visible change directly or obscure it temporarily through overlapping system effects.

Intake drift introduces another layer of complexity because small changes can accumulate gradually without dramatic awareness. Intake structure may appear broadly similar while portions slowly increase, convenience eating becomes more common, reactive eating rises, reward responsiveness intensifies, or eating frequency shifts subtly across time. These changes are often interpreted morally, but the systems view is more precise. Intake drift is not proof of weak discipline or failure. It is one of several variables that may influence the storage–release balance as compensation pressure rises or fatigue accumulates.

The subtlety matters because visible plans are often evaluated categorically rather than dynamically. A person may feel they are "doing the same thing" because the general structure remains familiar, even while the actual intake environment has shifted modestly underneath. These shifts may narrow the original deficit gap gradually rather than through one obvious behavioral change.

Output reduction creates similar confusion because visible exercise can remain stable while total daily demand quietly declines. Chapter

15 established that energy demand includes more than formal workouts alone. Walking, posture energy, fidgeting, spontaneous movement, task effort, training intensity, work tolerance, and ordinary physical engagement all contribute to total output across time.

A plateau may therefore emerge even when planned exercise appears unchanged because hidden output has narrowed underneath the visible routine. There may be more sitting, less pacing, slower movement, lower posture energy, reduced training quality, less spontaneous activity, shorter tolerance for effort, or lower willingness to initiate movement. These shifts often occur gradually and without deliberate intention. The visible workout remains present, but the broader release-and-use environment becomes smaller.

Adaptation adds another layer because the system itself changes under sustained deficit pressure. Chapter 11 explained that as body mass declines and reduced availability persists, the original energy gap may narrow. A smaller body generally requires less energy to maintain than a larger body. Output may become more efficient. Recovery allocation may shift. Spontaneous movement may decline. The same visible structure may therefore produce slower visible change later because the conditions are no longer identical to those present at the beginning.

This does not mean the earlier deficit was imaginary. It means the system adapted around sustained constraint. The plateau may therefore reflect a genuine slowing of visible change caused by altered conditions rather than by failure or system collapse.

Measurement noise further complicates interpretation because biological systems do not produce perfectly smooth visible outputs. Day-to-day fluctuations are normal. Short observation windows are inherently noisy. A flat sequence of readings may partly reflect the limitations of measurement itself rather than a complete absence of underlying change.

This becomes especially important because the scale compresses gradual biological processes into isolated numerical snapshots. Real physiology operates continuously across time, while measurement captures intermittent surface observations. Temporary flatness can therefore emerge even when underlying movement remains active beneath the visible signal.

Plateaus often create panic precisely because the visible signal feels definitive. When visible change slows or disappears temporarily, interpretation tends to move rapidly toward failure language. The mind assumes the system has stopped responding, that progress is gone, or that something has become fundamentally wrong. The plateau becomes emotionally interpreted as a dead end rather than analytically interpreted as ambiguous feedback.

This panic interpretation often arises because visible outputs are treated as complete explanations rather than partial observations. If the scale is assumed to represent fat mass directly and perfectly, then visible flatness appears to prove that no underlying change exists. But the earlier mechanisms in this book repeatedly point toward a different conclusion. Fat loss occurs within a dynamic system shaped by storage pressure, release-and-use pressure, appetite compensation, adaptation, recovery demand, glucose behavior, output tolerance, stress load, and measurement variability. Visible outcomes compress all of those interacting processes into a limited outward signal.

A plateau may therefore reflect several different situations operating underneath the same visible surface. In some cases, visible slowing is genuine. The rate of change has truly decreased because adaptation has narrowed the original gap, output has declined, intake has drifted upward, or recovery conditions have changed. In other situations, underlying fat loss may still be occurring while water retention, glycogen shifts, digestive contents, or recovery-related fluid behavior obscure the visible signal temporarily. In many cases, several variables are moving simultaneously, creating ambiguity that makes short-term interpretation difficult.

This distinction matters because visible flatness and biological stasis are not identical. A flatter visible signal does not prove that nothing is happening underneath. It means the visible signal has become harder to read clearly across that interval.

The interpretive task of the chapter therefore shifts away from verdict language and toward systems interpretation. The plateau itself is not the mechanism. It is the visible expression through which multiple possible mechanisms may be appearing simultaneously.

This relationship is best understood through the Plateau Feedback Mechanism.

Plateau Feedback Mechanism: A plateau signals that visible change has slowed, stopped, or become masked by other variables.

The mechanism contains three interpretive sides operating together. The first is visible slowdown. The observable outcome becomes flatter, slower, or less responsive than expected. The second is possible hidden causes. Water retention, glycogen shifts, digestive contents, stress load, adaptation, intake drift, output reduction, inflammation-related fluid behavior, and measurement noise may all contribute to the visible plateau. The third is interpretive uncertainty. The visible signal alone does not identify which mechanism is dominant underneath the surface.

The purpose of the mechanism is not to prescribe a fix. It is to provide a more accurate interpretation of what the visible plateau actually represents.

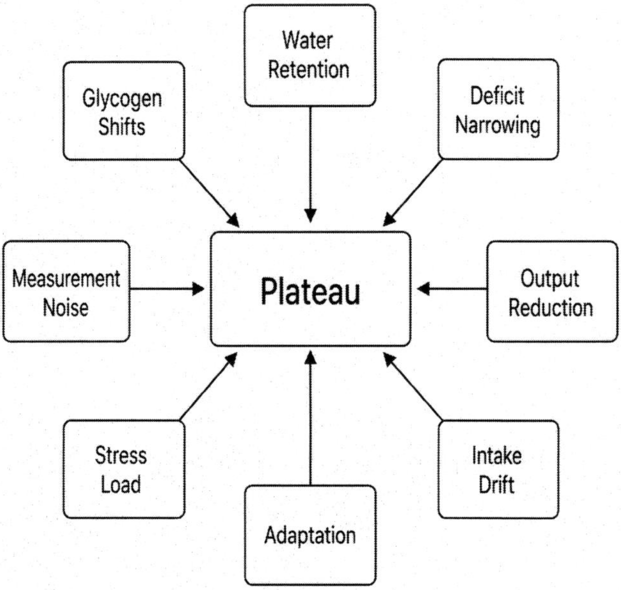

[Figure 16: Plateau Sources Map]

The figure places the visible plateau at the center while multiple surrounding variables feed into it simultaneously. Water retention, glycogen shifts, digestive contents, intake drift, output reduction, adaptation, stress load, and measurement noise all point toward the same visible observation. The structure of the figure matters because it prevents the plateau itself from being mistaken for the cause. The plateau is the outward signal. The surrounding mechanisms represent some of the underlying processes capable of shaping that signal.

The diagram also reinforces why short-term interpretation becomes difficult during stalled periods. Multiple variables may overlap at once. A person may simultaneously experience modest intake drift, higher recovery strain, increased water retention, lower spontaneous movement, and ordinary measurement variability while still maintaining some degree of underlying stored-energy reduction. The visible signal compresses those interacting layers into one outward observation, which is why isolated stalls often appear more definitive than they actually are.

This matters because interpretation shapes the meaning assigned to the experience. If the plateau is interpreted as direct proof of failure, the response often becomes panic, escalation, overcorrection, or aggressive troubleshooting. Ordinary variability becomes pathologized. Temporary ambiguity becomes evidence that nothing is working. The visible signal is treated as absolute rather than conditional.

A systems-oriented interpretation produces a calmer and more precise conclusion. The visible signal has become less clear. Several variables may be contributing simultaneously. The plateau does not automatically identify which mechanism is dominant underneath, nor does it automatically prove that all underlying progress has stopped.

This broader interpretive frame becomes increasingly important over longer time horizons because fat loss is not expressed through perfectly linear visible change. The visible signal fluctuates. Water compartments shift. Output changes. Recovery status changes. Appetite pressure changes. Stress accumulates and resolves. Measurement noise persists. Short-term observations therefore contain ambiguity that cannot always be resolved immediately through the visible signal alone.

Chapter 17 will widen the frame further by examining long-term trend interpretation. Once plateaus are understood as ambiguous feedback rather than final verdicts, isolated stalls become easier to interpret within larger patterns across time. Fat loss is not best understood through single weigh-ins or short windows of visible flatness. It is better understood through broader directional trends unfolding across a continuously changing system.

A plateau is therefore not always a stop signal. Often it is an interpretive signal that visible change has slowed, become obscured, or become temporarily harder to read clearly while multiple underlying processes continue moving underneath the surface.

Rebound and Return Pressure

Chapter 16 explained that plateaus are often misread because visible signals do not automatically explain the mechanisms underneath them. A flatter scale trend may reflect water retention, glycogen shifts, digestive contents, intake drift, output reduction, stress load, adaptation, or measurement ambiguity rather than a complete stop in stored-energy change. The same interpretive discipline becomes necessary after fat loss has occurred. Rebound is commonly interpreted as proof of failure, but the systems view is more precise. Regain after loss often reflects return pressure acting on a system that has not yet stabilized around its new condition.

This distinction matters because fat loss is frequently treated as though the process ends once a visible target has been reached. The visible reduction becomes the finish line, and maintenance is assumed to occur automatically afterward. But the biological conditions that produced loss do not instantly disappear once the visible outcome changes. Appetite pressure, adaptation, lower output, stress load, environmental friction, altered energy requirements, and prior behavior patterns may still remain active after visible reduction has occurred.

Rebound is therefore best understood not as a moral collapse, but as movement back toward prior storage levels when return pressure exceeds the stability of the new pattern. That movement may appear through gradual weight regain, rising appetite pressure, reduced output, increasing intake, re-emergence of prior routines, or restoration of older energy patterns. Rebound is not inevitable, but it is understandable within a system attempting to re-establish continuity after a period of altered energy balance.

The distinction between fat loss and maintenance becomes important here because they are not identical physiological states. Fat loss occurs during periods in which release-and-use pressure exceeds storage pressure strongly enough for stored reserves to decline across time. Maintenance represents a different condition. Maintenance requires a new equilibrium in which intake, output, appetite, recovery, environment, and daily behavior can hold the newer storage level without ongoing instability or escalating compensation.

Reaching a lower weight or lower stored-fat level therefore does not automatically mean the system has stabilized around that condition. The visible outcome may change before the surrounding system fully reorganizes around it. This creates what can be understood as a transition gap: the unstable period between active loss and durable stability.

During this transition gap, the system may still carry many of the pressures that developed during fat loss itself. Appetite signals may remain elevated. Output may still be lower than before. Recovery burden may remain high. Stress load may still interfere with stability. Familiar environmental cues may continue pulling behavior toward older patterns. The visible outcome has changed, but the surrounding behavioral and physiological environment may not yet support that outcome reliably.

This unstable middle phase is where rebound pressure often becomes most visible. The person may no longer be actively pursuing further loss, but the new condition has not yet become fully durable. The earlier structure that supported reduction may loosen before a stable replacement pattern has formed. Return pressure begins filling the gap.

Appetite pressure remains one of the strongest contributors because the system may continue responding to reduced reserves, altered availability, prior deficit exposure, and changing body mass even after visible loss has occurred. Hunger does not automatically normalize the moment a lower weight is reached. Cravings, food focus, urgency, and reduced satiety may continue for some period because the system is still interpreting reduced reserves and altered energy conditions relative to its prior state.

This is especially important because appetite pressure after loss is often interpreted psychologically rather than regulatorily. Increased hunger is treated as lack of discipline or fading motivation instead of being understood as ongoing biological pressure toward restored availability. But the system does not recognize the visible outcome as a symbolic endpoint. It continues regulating based on availability, stored reserves, energy demand, stress load, recovery status, and environmental exposure.

Reduced satiety can also persist into the post-loss period. Meals that once felt sufficiently satisfying may produce shorter-lasting fullness. Food focus may remain elevated. Eating may continue feeling mentally prominent because the earlier deficit period altered the broader appetite environment. These signals are not evidence that the person failed to "adapt mentally" to the new weight. They are part of the ongoing regulatory environment surrounding a system that recently experienced sustained reduction pressure.

Lower body mass introduces another layer because a smaller body generally requires less energy to maintain than a larger one. The post-loss environment is therefore not identical to the pre-loss environment even if the visible lifestyle appears similar. Returning to prior intake patterns after body mass has declined may increase storage pressure more easily because the system being maintained has changed.

This shift is often overlooked because people frequently compare post-loss conditions to earlier periods without accounting for altered maintenance requirements. The earlier intake pattern may have existed alongside greater body mass, higher spontaneous output, different appetite conditions, or different demand levels. Once body mass declines, the overall energy environment changes with it.

Reduced output can further increase rebound pressure because hidden demand often narrows during and after fat loss. Chapter 15 explained that total energy demand includes more than planned exercise alone. Spontaneous movement, posture energy, walking, fidgeting, task effort, training quality, work tolerance, and ordinary physical engagement all contribute to total output across time.

These outputs may remain suppressed after loss has occurred. A person may continue exercising formally while total daily movement stays lower than before. Fatigue may shorten tolerance for activity. Training intensity may drift downward. More sitting may replace earlier movement patterns. Recovery burden may remain elevated. These changes can quietly reduce release-and-use pressure even while the visible structure appears stable.

Adaptation also continues influencing the post-loss environment. Chapter 11 explained that sustained deficit pressure can narrow the original energy gap through increased efficiency, lower expenditure, and altered output patterns. These adaptations do not necessarily disappear immediately after visible reduction occurs. The system may remain more conservative, more efficient, or more responsive to changes in availability for some period afterward.

This should not be interpreted as metabolic damage or permanent impairment. It is better understood as continued adjustment within a system that recently operated under sustained energy constraint. The same adaptive processes that helped preserve continuity during fat loss may continue influencing maintenance stability afterward.

Stress load compounds these pressures because stress affects multiple regulatory layers simultaneously. Appetite pressure may rise under higher stress conditions. Sleep disruption may increase fatigue and food urgency. Recovery quality may decline. Glucose volatility may intensify cravings and reactive eating pressure. Output tolerance may narrow. Environmental friction may become harder to absorb.

These overlapping pressures matter because maintenance stability depends partly on whether the newer pattern can continue functioning under ordinary life conditions rather than only under tightly controlled conditions. If stress consistently increases appetite, reduces output, disrupts recovery, and raises eating pressure while the new pattern remains fragile, return pressure grows stronger.

Environment matters for similar reasons because behavior occurs inside physical and social contexts rather than in isolation. Food availability, convenience exposure, work schedules, travel, family patterns, social eating, emotional strain, and routine disruption all shape the pressure environment surrounding eating and movement behavior.

Old patterns often remain deeply connected to ordinary surroundings. Familiar restaurants, evening routines, work habits, convenience foods, social rituals, or stress-associated eating patterns may still exist unchanged after fat loss occurs. The newer pattern must therefore operate inside an environment partly built around older routines and older forms of stability.

This connects directly to habit patterns, which frequently re-emerge during the transition gap because familiar behavior requires less effort to execute. Previous meal timing, portion norms, convenience choices, evening eating patterns, stress responses, activity habits, and environmental reactions may remain neurologically and behaviorally well established even after visible loss occurs.

Under fatigue, stress, or reduced recovery capacity, familiar pathways often become easier to resume because they demand less conscious regulation. This does not mean the person secretly wanted to fail. It reflects the reality that older behavior patterns were previously stabilized across long periods of repetition. The system often drifts toward what is familiar when newer patterns remain fragile or effort-intensive.

Maintenance instability emerges when the newer intake, output, recovery, appetite, and environmental pattern has not yet become durable enough to support the lower storage level consistently. This distinction matters because maintenance failure is often interpreted personally rather than structurally. The person is blamed instead of the stability environment being examined.

But the systems perspective frames the issue differently. The newer pattern did not yet stabilize strongly enough to hold against the combined pressures of appetite, adaptation, reduced output, stress, environmental exposure, and prior behavioral pathways. The visible regain reflects a mismatch between return pressure and stabilization capacity rather than a collapse of character.

Return pressure develops from both intake-side and output-side mechanisms simultaneously. Intake pressure may rise through hunger, cravings, food focus, environmental exposure, reward sensitivity, convenience eating, and habit return. Output pressure may narrow through lower movement, fatigue, reduced spontaneous activity, lower posture energy, reduced work tolerance, or declining training quality. Together, these shifts gradually move the storage–release balance back toward storage.

Importantly, rebound is often gradual rather than dramatic. Popular narratives frequently portray regain as a sudden collapse, but system behavior is usually slower and more cumulative. Slightly larger portions, less movement, reduced recovery, increasing convenience eating, more fatigue, or declining attention to the newer structure may accumulate quietly across time.

The gradual nature of rebound matters because it reinforces why moral interpretation becomes misleading. Small environmental and behavioral drifts occur inside a changing physiological system carrying adaptation, appetite pressure, stress load, and altered output. The regain pathway therefore develops through accumulating pressure rather than through one singular moment of failure.

This entire process can be understood through the Return Pressure Mechanism.

Return Pressure Mechanism: After loss, multiple signals and behaviors can push the system back toward prior storage levels unless the new pattern stabilizes.

The mechanism contains three interacting sides. The first is the post-loss state. Body mass is lower, energy requirements have changed, prior deficit exposure may still influence appetite and output, and adaptation may still shape efficiency and recovery allocation. The second side is return pressure itself. Hunger, cravings, reduced satiety, lower output, fatigue, environmental exposure, habit return, stress load, and behavioral drift all increase pressure toward restored availability and prior stability patterns. The third side is stabilization requirement. The newer pattern must become durable enough to continue functioning without excessive strain despite these overlapping pressures.

The mechanism does not imply rebound is guaranteed. It means rebound risk increases when return pressure exceeds the stability of the newer pattern.

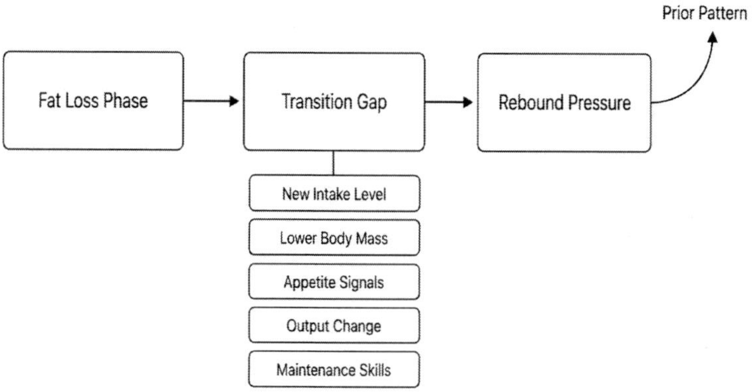

[Figure 17: Fat Loss → Transition Gap → Rebound Pressure]

The figure presents fat loss achievement on the left, followed by a central transition gap rather than an immediate stable endpoint. From that transition zone, multiple pressures branch outward: appetite pressure, lower output, habit return, stress and environmental exposure, and increasing storage pressure. These pressures then converge toward rebound pressure.

The structure of the figure matters because it prevents regain from being interpreted as a single behavioral failure. The transition gap is unstable precisely because multiple regulatory and environmental forces remain active simultaneously while the new pattern is still consolidating. The figure also emphasizes that rebound pressure emerges gradually through overlapping influences rather than through one isolated cause.

The side note that stability requires a new pattern to hold is equally important. Visible loss alone is not synonymous with long-term stability. The surrounding intake, output, recovery, appetite, environmental, and behavioral systems must also reorganize around the newer condition strongly enough to resist return pressure across time.

This broader interpretation changes how regain itself is understood. If rebound is framed as moral failure, then the same panic language that surrounded plateaus reappears. The visible regain becomes proof that the effort "didn't work," that the person lacked discipline, or that the earlier loss was somehow illegitimate.

A systems interpretation reaches a different conclusion. Rebound indicates that the pressures pulling toward prior stability became stronger than the system's ability to maintain the newer condition. Appetite, output, recovery, stress, environment, adaptation, and behavioral familiarity all continued influencing the post-loss environment after the visible reduction phase ended.

This perspective also explains why rebound can occur even after substantial success. The visible outcome may have changed dramatically while the surrounding regulatory and behavioral systems changed more slowly. If the newer pattern remains fragile, ordinary life pressures gradually expose the instability underneath it.

The larger implication is that fat loss cannot be understood purely as a temporary reduction event detached from long-term system organization. The ability to lose stored energy and the ability to stabilize around a newer condition are related but distinct processes. One concerns reduction pressure. The other concerns whether the broader system can hold the newer state without escalating compensation or increasing return pressure.

Chapter 18 will widen this frame further by shifting from temporary reduction toward long-term stability itself. The endpoint is not merely visible loss. The deeper question is whether the system can continue operating around the newer condition without constant escalation, rigid control, or persistent instability. Long-term stability depends not only on creating reduction pressure, but on whether the surrounding intake, output, recovery, appetite, environmental, and behavioral systems become durable enough to support the newer pattern across time.

Rebound is therefore not proof of weakness. It is a sign that the forces pulling toward prior stability became stronger than the new pattern's ability to hold against them.

Fat Loss Stability as an Outcome, Not a Target

This book has not treated fat loss as a simple act of subtraction. Across the preceding chapters, fat loss has been reframed as a regulated stored-energy process occurring inside a larger metabolic system. Visible change may be the part most easily noticed, but visible change is not the full mechanism. Stored reserves decline only when access, mobilization, utilization, storage pressure, release pressure, appetite, demand, recovery, adaptation, and compensation remain organized enough across time for reduction to continue without overwhelming system continuity.

Fat loss is often treated as a target because it is visible, measurable, and culturally emphasized. It can be tracked, compared, named, and judged. This visibility gives fat loss a sense of authority that many internal processes do not have. But visibility does not make it the body's highest biological priority. The body is not organized around producing visible reduction. It is organized around maintaining function under changing conditions.

The deeper priorities of the system are continuity, energy availability, tissue function, glucose regulation, recovery, movement capacity, appetite signaling, stress response, sleep stability, adaptation, and survival across time. Fat loss may occur within that system, but it does not outrank the system. Stored energy can decline when conditions support release and use, but the body must still maintain circulation, cognition, repair, temperature regulation, immune activity, movement, and daily function while that reduction occurs.

This is why fat loss cannot be understood accurately as a direct reward for effort, discipline, or arithmetic alone. It is not merely the disappearance of stored tissue. It is the outcome of a coordinated sequence. Body fat first had to be understood as stored energy and reserve capacity rather than as passive excess. Stored energy then had to become accessible. Access was not automatic, because reserves are regulated according to feeding state, insulin tone, stress, sleep, glycogen status, activity demand, and broader hormonal context.

After access comes mobilization, but mobilization is not completion. Stored fat can be released from storage and still fail to become meaningful reduction if it is not used. Released energy can circulate, be displaced by other fuels, or return toward storage depending on demand, fuel availability, insulin signaling, metabolic flexibility, stress load, and recovery state. Fat loss becomes meaningful only when mobilized energy continues into utilization strongly enough across time to reduce the reserve.

Utilization completes that early pathway. Released energy must be taken up and used by tissues. It needs a destination. Demand from movement, organ function, thermoregulation, cognition, tissue repair, immune activity, posture, work tolerance, and daily function helps determine whether mobilized energy becomes functional output. Without utilization, release remains an incomplete event.

The storage–release balance then places the pathway into a longer time frame. Fat loss does not require storage to disappear completely. Storage remains normal. Release remains normal. The body continues storing, releasing, circulating, and using energy across changing conditions. Fat loss occurs when release and use exceed storage and re-storage over time. The question is not whether storage ever occurs, but whether the long-term balance favors reduction of the stored reserve.

Regulation shapes that balance. Insulin is one major signal in this process, but it is not an enemy and not a single controller. It helps coordinate incoming energy, nutrient uptake, storage, fuel partitioning, and access to stored reserves. Higher insulin tone generally supports incoming energy handling and reduced reliance on long-term reserves. Lower insulin tone may permit greater access under some conditions. But insulin does not act alone.

Broader hormonal coordination shapes the same environment. Stress-related signaling, thyroid-related signaling, hunger and satiety signals, reproductive signaling, sleep-related regulation, and nervous system state all influence energy availability, appetite pressure, demand, recovery, throughput, and reserve protection. Fat loss is not governed by one hormone or one switch. It emerges within coordinated signaling across multiple systems.

The deficit signal then explains why energy balance matters without reducing the body to a spreadsheet. A calorie deficit matters because stored reserves cannot decline meaningfully if incoming energy and energy returning to storage consistently exceed release and use. But the deficit is not self-executing. Reduced incoming energy becomes biologically meaningful when the system interprets it and responds through appetite, output, stored-energy access, mobilization, recovery, stress signaling, and adaptation.

When that signal persists, the system adapts. Adaptation is not damage. It is adjustment under repeated energy constraint. Lower body mass changes energy requirements. Output may decline. Movement may become less spontaneous. Efficiency may increase. Appetite pressure may rise. Recovery may become harder to support. The original gap that supported fat loss can narrow because the system has changed.

Compensation follows as return pressure. Reduced energy availability can increase hunger, cravings, food focus, fatigue, lower movement, reduced output, and behavioral drift. These responses are not character flaws. They are regulatory pressures that can push the system back toward prior stability. Fat loss stability depends on whether these pressures remain coordinated enough that reduction can continue without compensation becoming dominant.

Appetite pressure is one of the most important behavioral surfaces of that regulation. Hunger, satiety loss, cravings, food urgency, reward sensitivity, and food focus translate internal energy conditions into signals that influence behavior. Appetite is not merely preference, and it is not evidence of weak control. It is the interface through which reduced availability, stress, sleep disruption, glucose volatility, recovery burden, and stored-energy change become behaviorally relevant.

Glucose volatility can amplify that pressure. Stable glucose does not guarantee fat loss, and unstable glucose does not make fat loss impossible. But volatility in glucose availability can increase hunger, fatigue, cravings, urgency, reactive eating pressure, and output instability. It affects the environment surrounding fat loss by making energy availability feel less stable and by increasing compensation pressure.

Energy demand forms the output side of the same system. Released energy needs a destination. Demand is not only formal exercise. Daily movement, posture, fidgeting, task effort, training quality, work tolerance, household movement, cognitive effort, and general function all shape the release-and-use environment. Demand supports fat loss most effectively when it remains present, tolerable, and sustainable. Excessive demand can increase compensation, while hidden output decline can narrow release-and-use pressure even when the visible plan appears unchanged.

Plateaus reveal why interpretation matters. A plateau is not automatically failure. Visible change may slow, stop, or become masked by water retention, glycogen shifts, digestive contents, recovery-related fluid shifts, intake drift, output reduction, adaptation, stress load, or measurement noise. A plateau is feedback that the visible signal has become harder to read clearly, not proof that nothing is happening underneath.

Rebound shows the same principle after loss has occurred. Rebound is not weakness. It is return pressure that can emerge when the new pattern has not stabilized. Appetite pressure, lower output, adaptation, stress load, environmental cues, old habits, changed energy requirements, and maintenance instability can push the system back toward prior storage levels. Fat loss and maintenance are related, but they are not the same state. The system must stabilize around the newer condition for the outcome to hold.

These mechanisms converge into the book's final model.

Fat Loss Stability Mechanism: Fat loss remains stable when stored-energy release, utilization, appetite, demand, recovery, and adaptation stay coordinated over time.

The mechanism has three integrated sides.

The first is the stored-energy pathway. Reserve energy must become accessible, mobilized, circulated, and used. Presence of stored energy is not enough. Release is not enough. Utilization across time is what turns stored-energy movement into meaningful reduction.

The second is the regulatory environment. Insulin signaling, broader hormonal coordination, deficit signaling, adaptation, compensation, appetite pressure, glucose behavior, stress load, and recovery state shape whether the stored-energy pathway remains stable or becomes constrained. These variables do not need to be perfect, but when they work strongly against one another, reduction becomes less stable.

The third is long-term stability. Demand, recovery, maintenance conditions, plateau interpretation, and rebound pressure determine whether the outcome can persist without constant escalation. Fat loss is not complete simply because visible loss occurred. It becomes stable only when the broader system can continue functioning around the newer pattern.

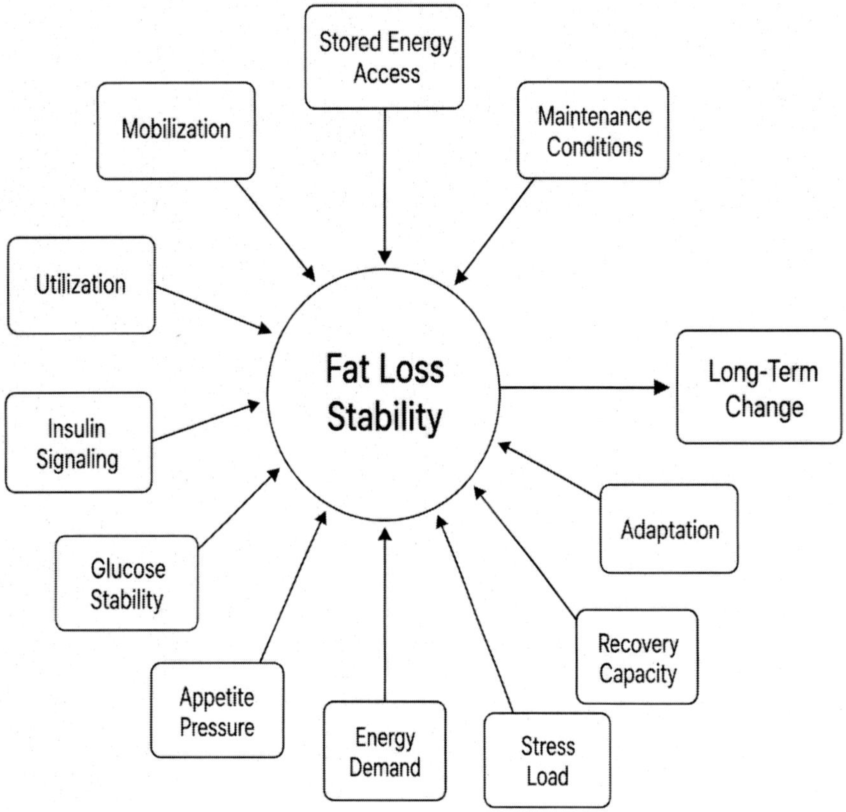

[Figure 18: Full Fat Loss Stability System Map]

The figure places fat loss stability at the center and surrounds it with the major systems developed throughout the book: stored energy access, mobilization, utilization, insulin signaling, hormonal coordination, deficit signal, adaptation, compensation, appetite pressure, glucose stability, energy demand, recovery, plateaus and feedback, and rebound pressure. The bottom note states that stability emerges from coordination over time.

This figure should not be read as a hierarchy with one master variable controlling the outcome. No single node governs fat loss stability by itself. Stored energy must become accessible and used, but appetite, demand, recovery, adaptation, glucose behavior, compensation, and return pressure determine whether the outcome remains stable across time. The map represents coordination rather than command.

This is why fat loss is better understood as an outcome than as a target. A target frame encourages the visible result to become the central measure of the system. Everything is judged by whether the number moves, how quickly it moves, and whether the visible reduction continues. An outcome frame places fat loss back inside the system that produces it. Fat loss becomes one possible expression of coordinated metabolic conditions rather than the highest purpose of metabolic health.

This protects the interpretation from diet-culture compression. The body is not failing when it prioritizes recovery, appetite signaling, energy availability, or function. The body is regulating. A system that cannot sleep, recover, move, think, regulate appetite, tolerate stress, maintain glucose stability, or preserve daily function may produce temporary loss, but temporary loss is not the same as stable loss.

Long-horizon function therefore matters more than short-term intensity. Fat loss produced under conditions that narrow recovery, raise compensation, increase fatigue, destabilize appetite, or amplify return pressure may become difficult to sustain even when visible reduction occurs. The system can be pushed into reduction without becoming stable around reduction.

Constraint awareness is part of accurate interpretation. Stress, poor sleep, reduced recovery capacity, high appetite pressure, glucose volatility, excessive demand, repeated restriction, and environmental friction can all narrow the conditions supporting stable fat loss. Recognizing constraints does not make the model pessimistic. It makes it accurate. Systems behave according to capacity, pressure, and feedback, not intention alone.

Maintenance completes the frame. Maintenance is not the passive aftermath of fat loss. It is the period in which the newer pattern must hold. The system must settle into a durable relationship among intake, output, appetite, recovery, demand, environment, and stored-energy regulation. Without that stabilization, return pressure can gradually move the system toward prior patterns.

This is why fat loss should not be treated as a permanent state of effort. A system cannot remain indefinitely organized around escalation, pressure, and reduction. Stable outcomes require conditions that can persist without continuously increasing strain. The endpoint is not more force. The endpoint is coordination strong enough that the newer pattern can remain compatible with function.

The central argument of the book resolves here.

Fat loss is not a switch. It is not a moral result. It is not the direct evidence of discipline. It is not the body's highest priority. It is a regulated outcome that can emerge when stored energy, access, release, use, appetite, demand, recovery, and adaptation remain aligned enough across time.

Fat loss stability is not achieved by forcing one variable harder.

It emerges when the system can continue functioning while stored energy, appetite, demand, recovery, and adaptation remain coordinated across time.

About the Author

Nathan Reed writes about metabolic stability in systems exposed to load, variability, and time.

His work examines how biological capacity is shaped by energy availability, recovery architecture, sleep amplitude, muscle mass, environmental demand and workload. Rather than treating nutrition, fasting, sleep, and training as isolated tactics, he approaches them as interacting regulatory systems governed by margin, buffering, oscillatory coherence, and constraint dominance.

The Stability framework explores how physiological compression accumulates gradually and how proportional calibration preserves long-horizon resilience across decades. The objective is not peak optimization, but preservation of functional continuity under load.

Fat Loss Stability is part of a broader metabolic stability ecosystem developed under Perennial Publishing, each volume addressing a distinct vector of biological durability.

The work is designed for readers who prefer structural clarity over motivational rhetoric and long-horizon coherence over short-term intensity.

The Metabolic Stability Series

Metabolic Stability – (Cornerstone Volume)

Fasting Fundamentals – (Foundational Volume)

Intermittent Fasting

Prolonged Fasting

Electrolytes

Insulin Stability

Glucose Stability

Metabolic Flexibility

Appetite Stability

Energy Stability

Blood Sugar Stability

Fat Loss Stability

Future Titles Include:

Fatigue Stability

Craving Stability

The Vitality Series:

Sleep and Recovery

Strength and Aging

Hormones & Sexual Health

Part of a Broader Stability Framework

The Metabolic Stability Series is part of a larger stability ecosystem published by Perennial Publishing.

Related domains include:

Money Stability — structural durability in financial systems

Career Stability — positioning, load tolerance, and transition resilience

Mental Stability — cognitive steadiness under pressure and uncertainty

Emotional Stability — regulatory steadiness in environments that do not slow down

Foundations — low-fragility life architecture

Vitality — energy, strength, and biological function across time

Each domain approaches stability as a structural problem: capacity versus load, buffering versus shock, governance versus drift. Together, they form a unified framework for long-horizon durability across the major systems that shape human trajectory.

About Perennial Publishing

Perennial Publishing produces practical systems guides for building stability in an unstable world.

Our books explore the foundations of long-term resilience across health, finance, career, and everyday decision-making. Each title focuses on clear frameworks, durable principles, and practical strategies that help readers build lasting stability rather than short-term fixes.

The Perennial catalog includes series on metabolic health, financial stability, career systems, and personal consistency. While each book stands on its own, they share a common goal: helping individuals create durable systems that support a stable and sustainable life.